MASTERCLASS:
GOING DOWN

WITH A TEXT BY
IAN CAMERON

EPS

Acknowledgments

Special thanks are due to all who have taken part in creating this book, but especially to Lynn Paula Russell whose wonderful drawings provide the main source of graphic illustration and to our two gorgeous photgraphic models Jo-May and Frankie.

THE *Erotic* Print Society
London 2004

THE *Erotic* Print Society
EPS, 17 Harwood Road
LONDON SW6 4QP

Orderline (UK only): 0871 7110 134
Fax: +44 (0)20 7736 6330
Email: eps@dawson-marketing.co.uk
Web: www.eroticprints.org

© 2004 MacHo Ltd, London UK
© 2004 Cross River Ltd.

Printed and bound in Spain by Gráficas Viking, Barcelona

ISBN : 1-904989-01-2

No part of this publication may be reproduced by any means without the express written permission of the Publishers. The moral right of the author/illustrators of the text and the images has been asserted.

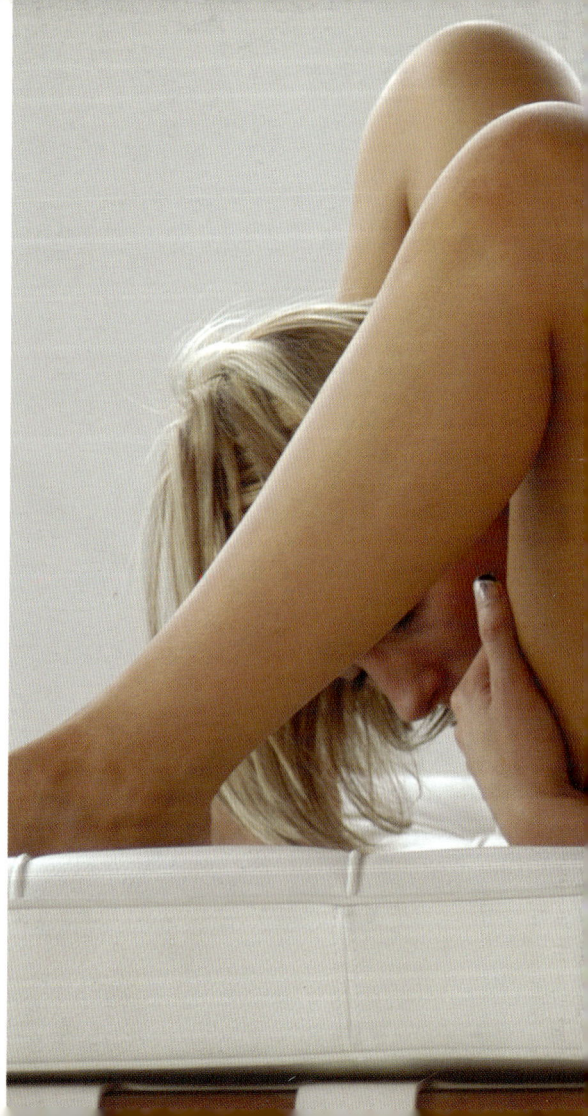

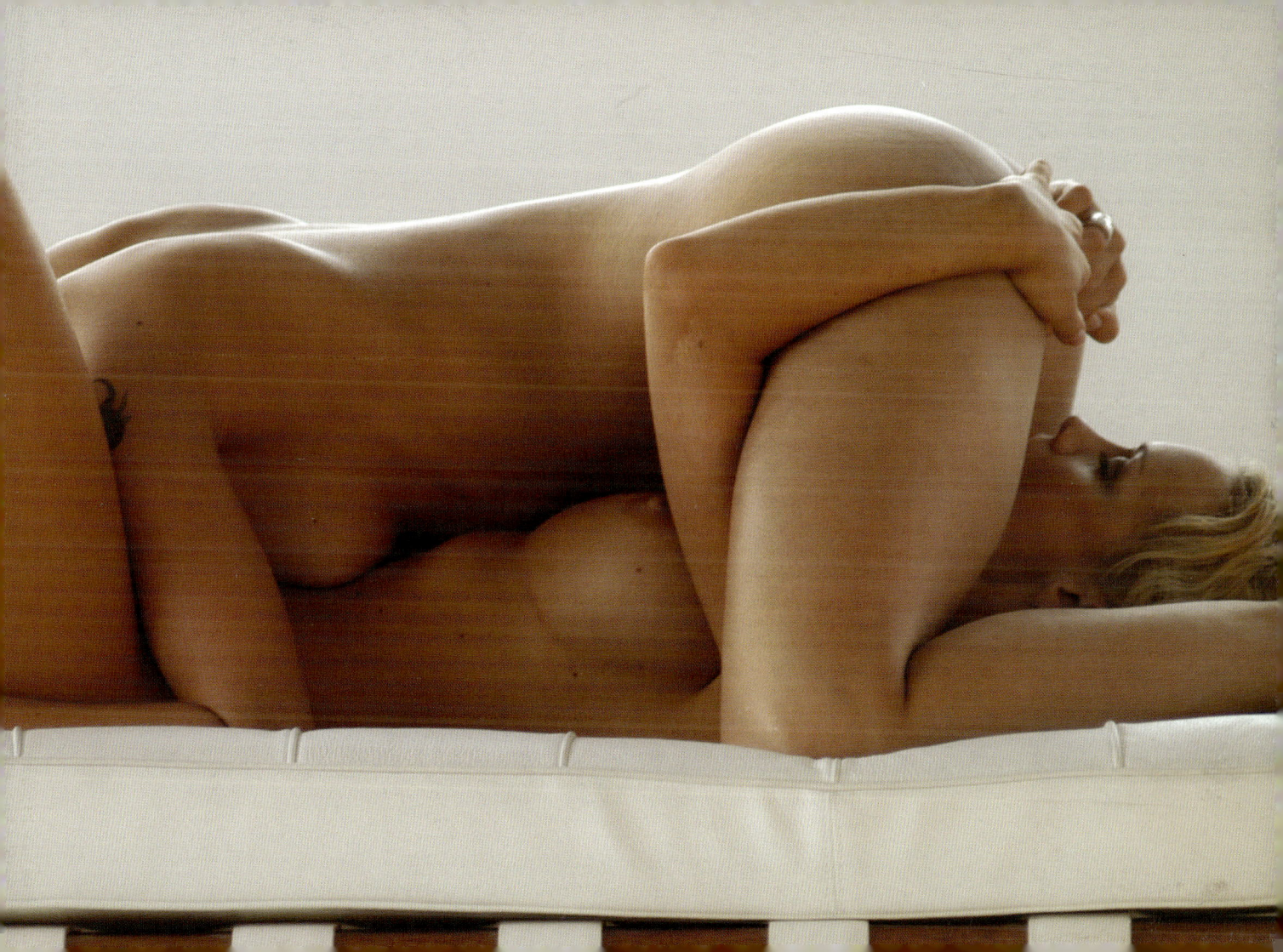

CONTENTS

	FOREWORD	*Page 7*
	INTRODUCTION	*Page 11*
I	**SECRETS OF FEMALE GENITAL ANATOMY (REVEALED)**	*Page 17*
II	**WHY SEX TIPS DON'T HELP**	*Page 27*
III	**STORYTELLING TECHNIQUES: THE OPENING SCENE**	*Page 35*
IV	**THE STORY CONTINUES**	*Page 41*
V	**HAND POSITIONS AND DEVICES**	*Page 47*
VI	**BODY POSITIONS**	*Page 65*
VII	**A WORD ABOUT HEALTH**	*Page 91*
	CONCLUSION	*Page 97*
	GALLERY, TERMS & INDEX	*Page 99*

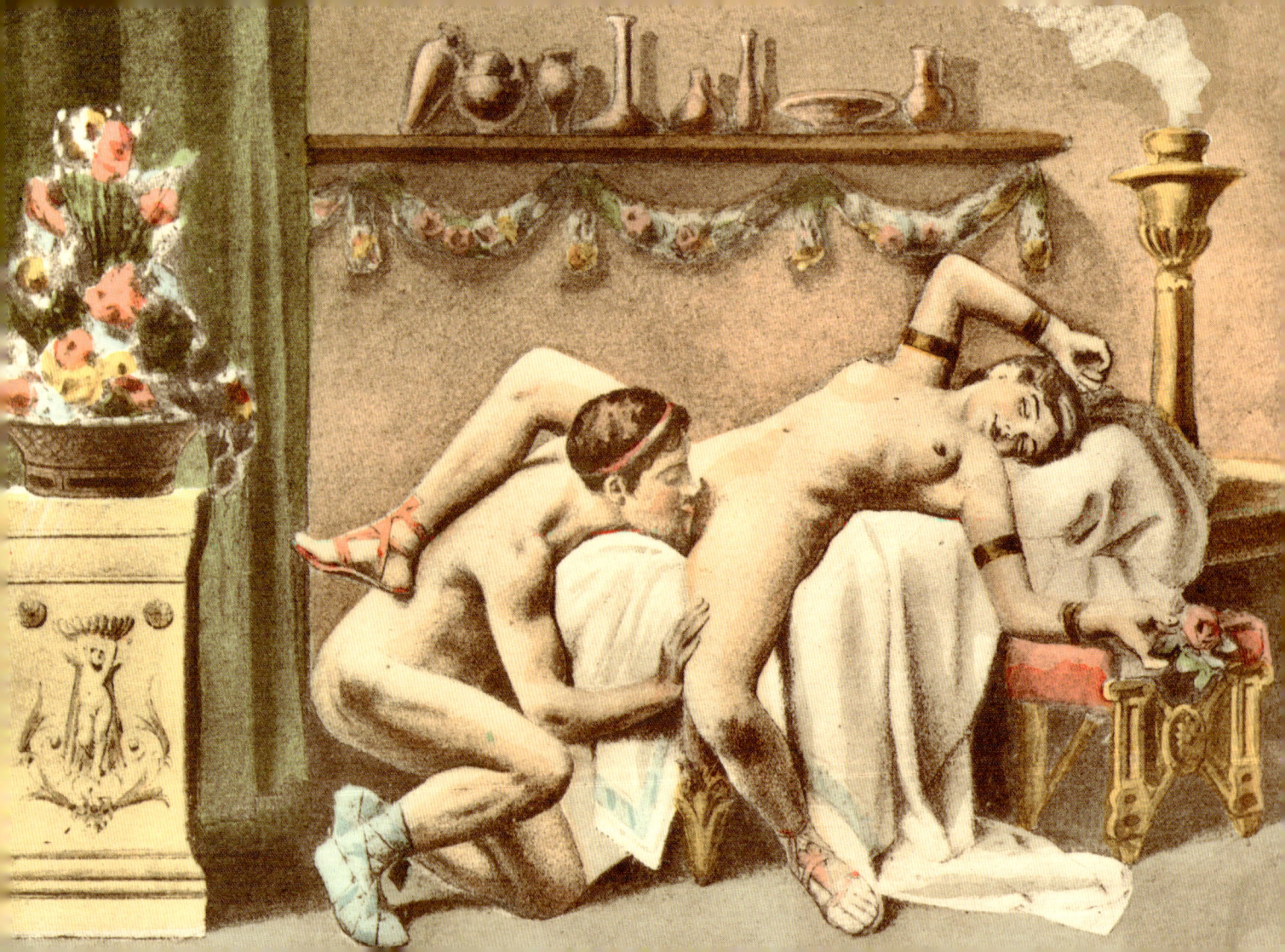

FOREWORD

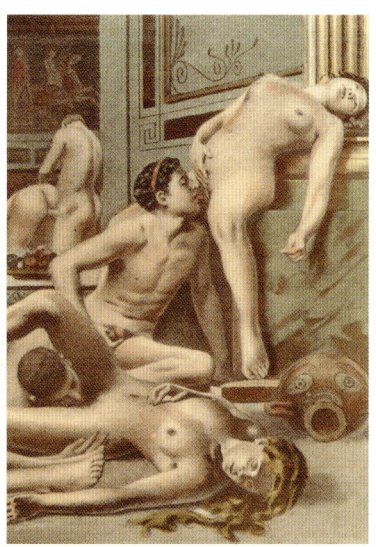 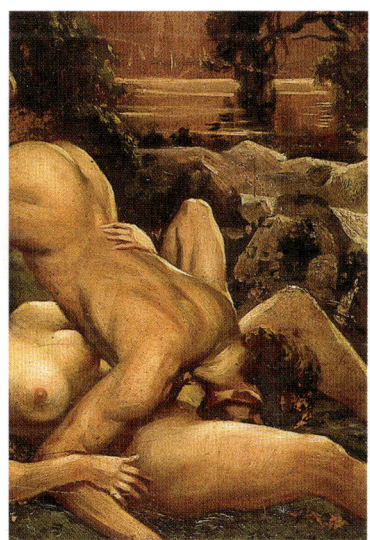

Cunnilingus. Surely there's nothing very special about a sex act that must have been around since the dawn of humanity? Wrong. There are some very special differences about this particular form of lovemaking. The lioness' share of sexual sensation and pleasure is with the female, not her male (or female) partner. And the act is in no way procreative: it is purely recreational (unless viewed in the context of foreplay for 'normal' sexual intercourse). And here is something else that makes it special and important: more women reach orgasm through this form of sex than any other.

Moreover it is the one sexual act between humans that combines male love with male heterosexual lust – where the male is, for once, acting relatively selflessly, and the female's enjoyment is paramount. So why - if going down on a woman arguably gives her greater pleasure and more orgasms than any other form of sex - do we tend to treat it as a second-class citizen?

Some men find it a worrying or even frightening experience, mainly through pure ignorance. Some see it as a necessary evil that will put his partner 'in a sexually receptive mood' before he can 'have his way'. Often a man's enjoyment of the act is usually

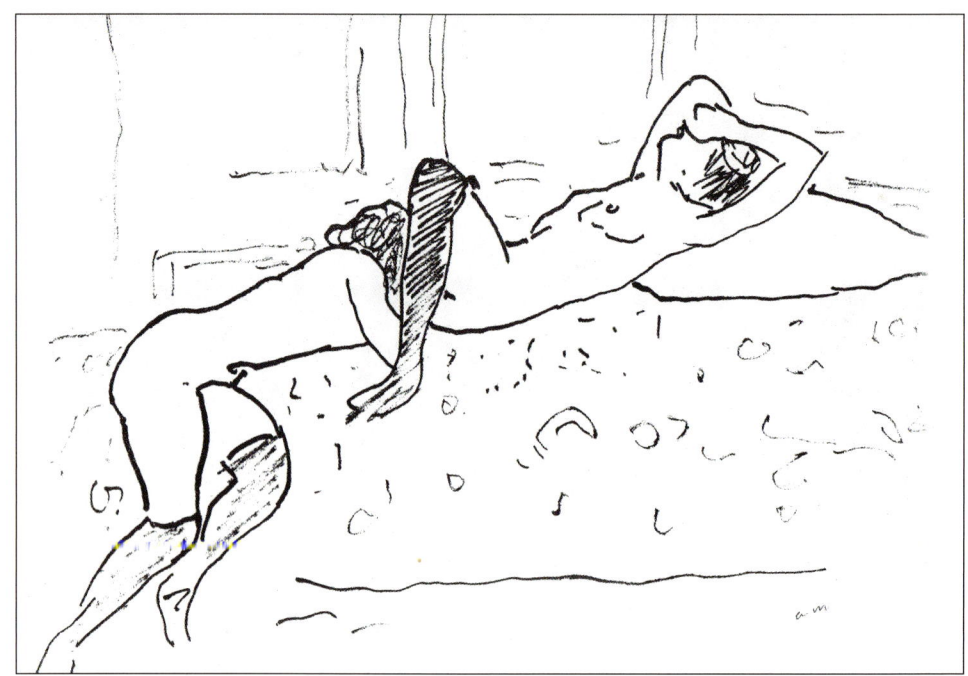

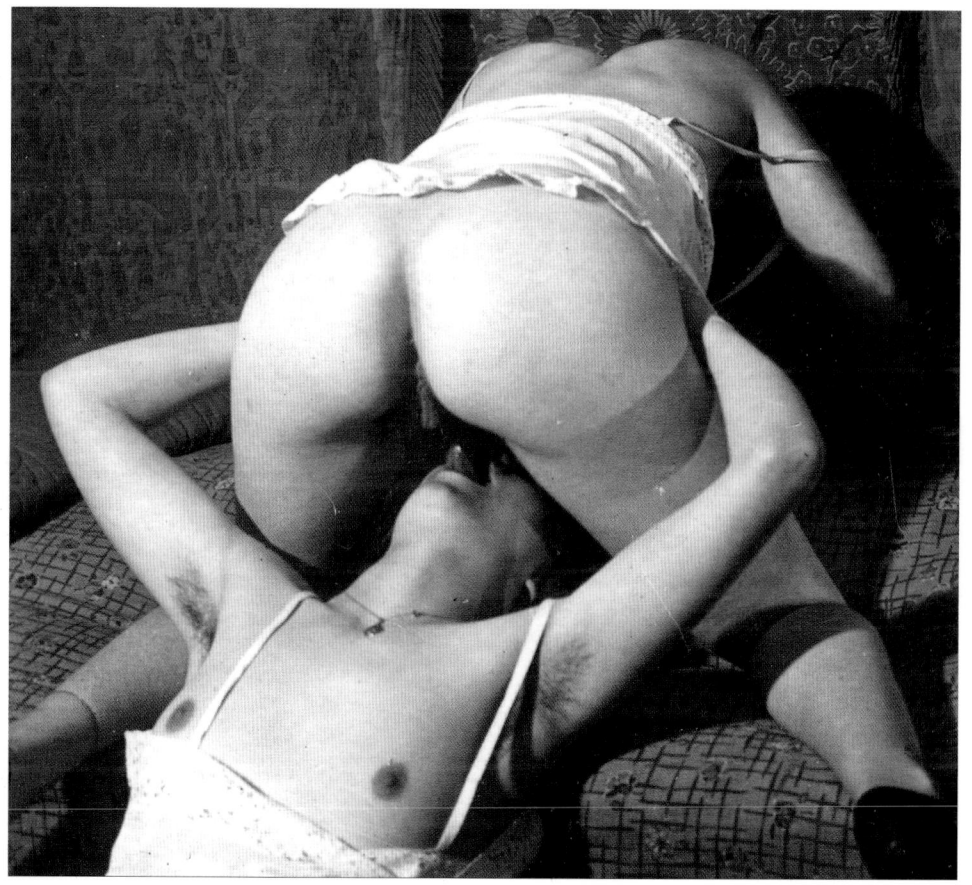

more cerebral than physical. Others see it as merely a means to an end, i.e. lubricating their partners and bringing them to approximately the same pitch of arousal as their own, in order to have penetrative sex with a greater degree of mutual enjoyment. And some men will find that going down is the most sexually exciting act that they can experience – preferable even to penetrative sex itself.

The dedicated cunnilinguist can unravel the mystery of a woman's genitals that in a way that a man who has only practiced penetrative sex, or very rudimentary oral sex, with a woman cannot. And he can make this voyage of discovery with the owner of the unknown territory herself. In Ian Cameron's inspirational text, readers will find much to demonstrate that going down is the most thrilling, the most rewarding and the noblest of sex acts. With his intuitive 'tongue talking' techniques, they are taken beyond the selfish limits of mere male sexual gratification and shown that cunnilingus is indeed the very threshold between pure lust and perfect love.

This is a book for the man or woman who would like to perfect their technique, for those would like to learn more, or even for those who consider themselves rank beginners. In return for a little sensitivity and patience – the rewards are incalculable.

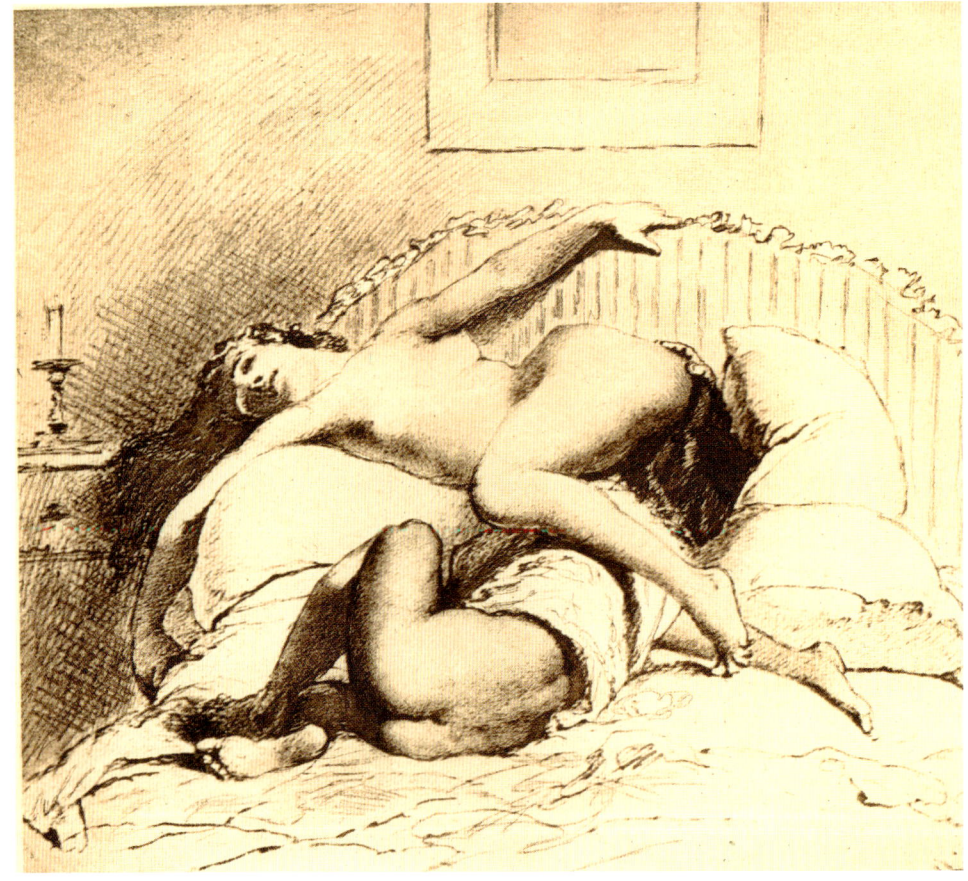

INTRODUCTION

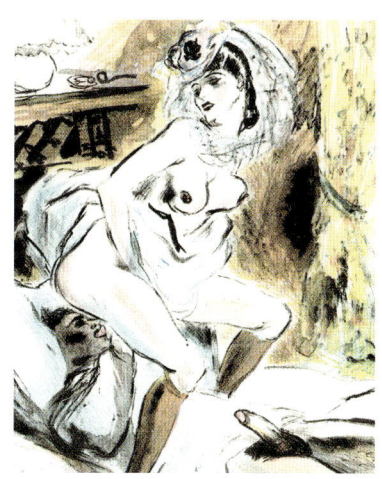 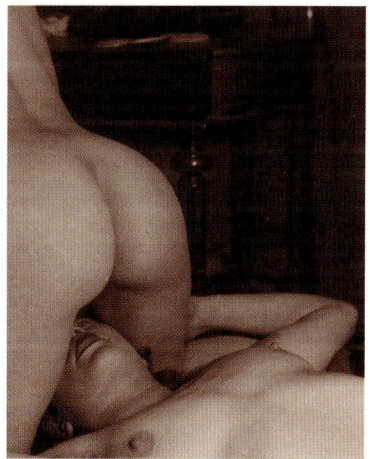

I n the spoof 50's science-fiction movie, *Earth Girls Are Easy*, a trio of aliens disguised as attractive young earth males are having a night out at a club. Drinks are served, and one of the aliens, forgetting his earth disguise, extends a two-foot long tongue into his glass. Seeing this, one of the young women present declares to her friends, "I'm going home with *him*."

For some reason we are all expected

to be born with certain abilities fully developed and functioning. Among these are a Sense Of Humour, Parenting, Relationships, and Sex. Especially sex.

This book is another small pebble on the how-to sex-book mountain. Its sub-heading could be Technique; its sub-sub heading Cunnilingus: the sexual stimulation of a woman's genitals with the lips and tongue. But as I hope to show, the dictionary definition is only half the story.

Physical technique is far from everything. Like many arts – and cunnilingus is an art – technique is as much mental as it is physical. And while art cannot be taught, a few tips and clues are all that's needed to put most people well on the way to producing consistently good art – as well as the occasional masterpiece.

Now the cliché is true: the primary

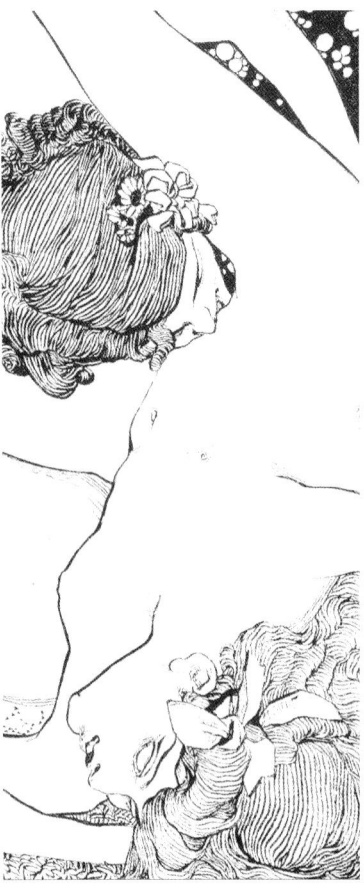

sex organ is between the ears (and no, it's not your nose); the way you think says as much about you as a cunning linguist as any acrobatics you can display with your lips and tongue.

Indeed, there is no better descriptive phrase for oral sex than "giving head." It's the head which does the giving. Your sexual creativity is inside your head, along with any other feelings you attach to it.

And if you think you're short on the creative – and everyone does at one time or another, no exceptions – this book will try to show you probably have more of that than you think.

Technique is of course useful if not essential, but above all it's the context in which the technique is used which marks out the cunnilingual artist from the sex-manual follower.

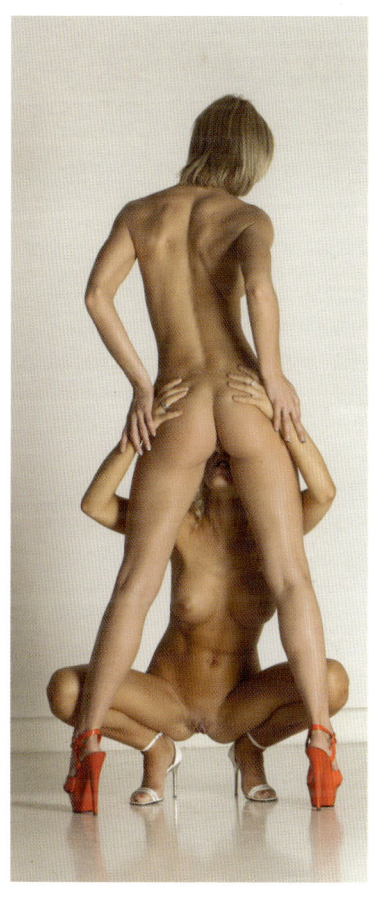
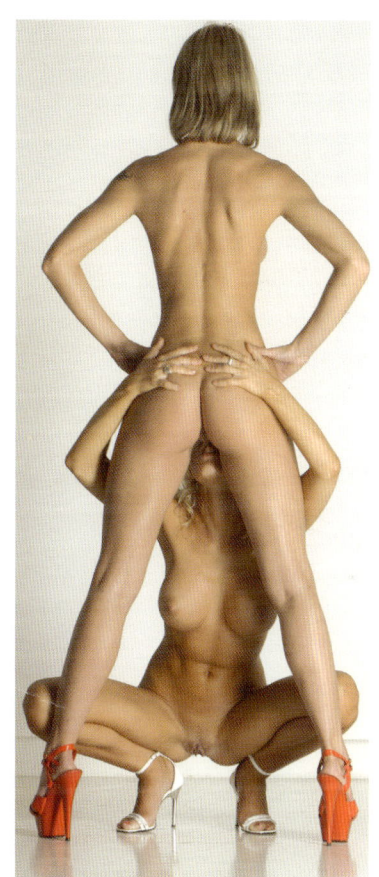
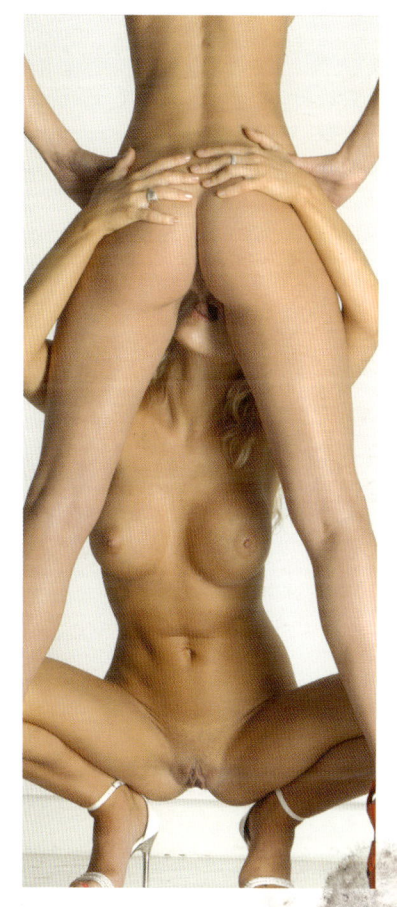

I make no apologies for leaving out references to feelings (tenderness, love, affection, etc.) except as they relate. Likewise to gender, except when it applies. I trust your ability to fit your feelings to the occasion, and in any case there are plenty of books around which claim to decode the shifting complexities of the human heart and instruct you as to their proper employment. This book will briefly cover three topics relative to the art of cunnilingual sex: the anatomical, the conceptual, and the technical. Understand the first, explore the second with the help of the third and your rewards will be many and memorable.

I freely admit the concept of 'Tongue Talking' is a bit unusual. Explaining the telling of a story sexually makes it difficult to separate each body part and give it its own list of techniques.

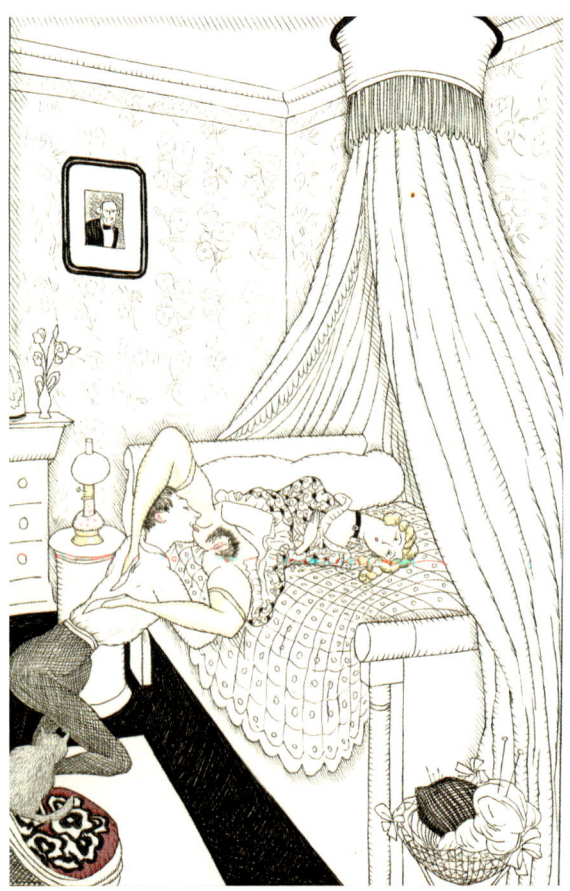

INSCRUTABLE PUSSY POWER

A CHINESE CONCUBINE of Emperors T'ai-tsung and Kao-tsung, named Wu Chao, reigned as empress. In 690 A.D. she removed the legitimate heir and took the throne herself under the name 'Emperor' Tse-t'ien. She even founded her own dynasty, disrupting the T'ang dynasty, calling it the Chou. It lasted for 15 years. During in this time she decreed that all visiting dignitaries should pay homage by performing cunnilingus on her; talk about sucking up to royalty...

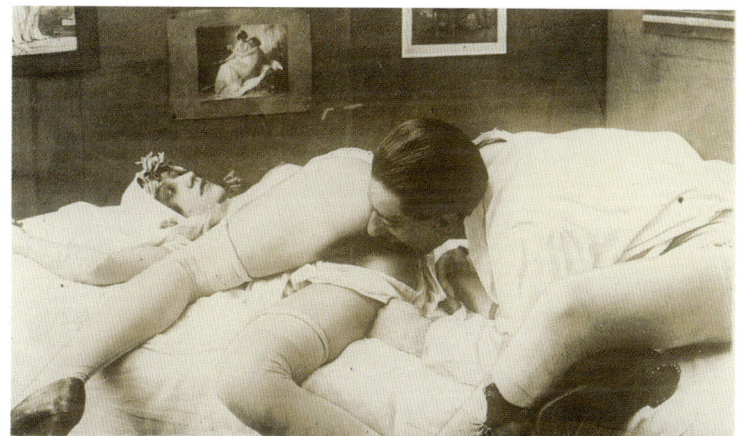

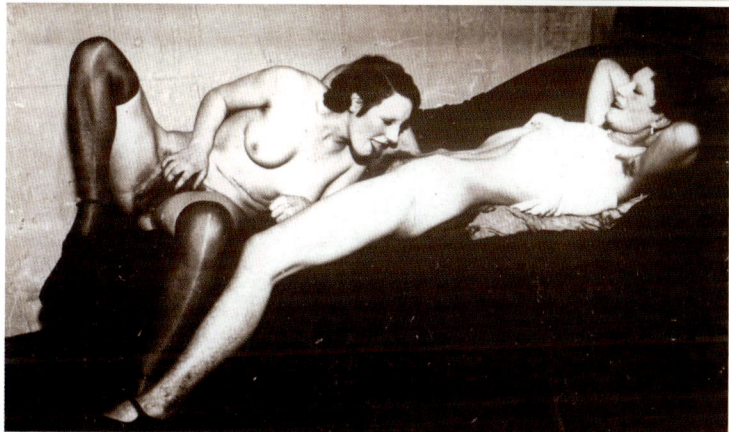

For those of you still impatient to fast-forward to the "hot tips" and still wonder what all the "story" business has to do with cunnilingus, let me ask you three questions: Do you go to a restaurant for dessert? Do you go into a movie at the end? Do you have sex in order to come? If the answer is "yes" to any of these, I suggest a medical check for Attention Deficit Disorder. Treatment is both available and effective.

What I have written could not have been achieved without the help and encouragement of my darling wife and our many enthusiastic friends, all experts in their own right, who have continued to furnish me with helpful contributions well past the deadline for the manuscript, for which I remain grateful.

IAN CAMERON

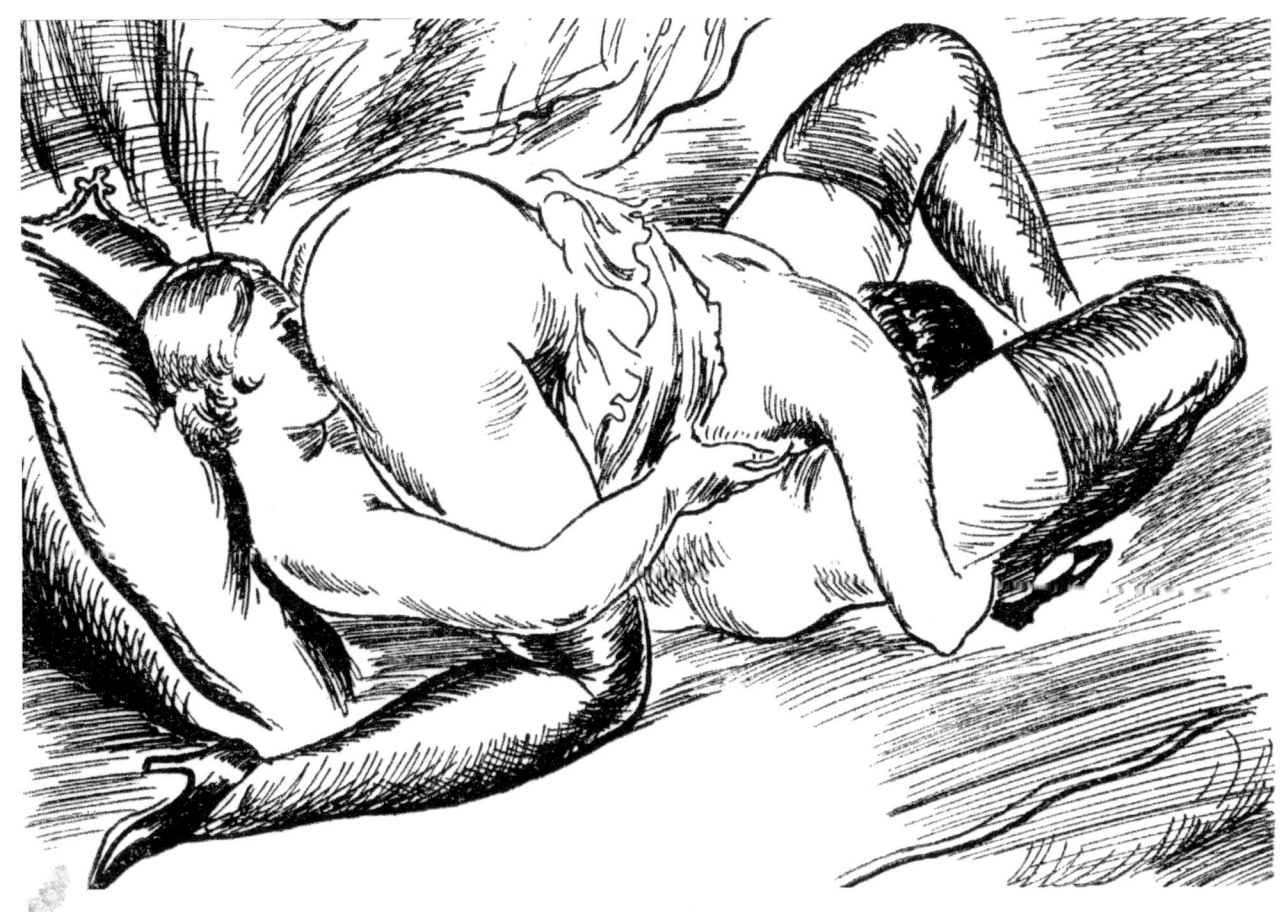

I   SECRETS OF FEMALE GENITAL ANATOMY (REVEALED)

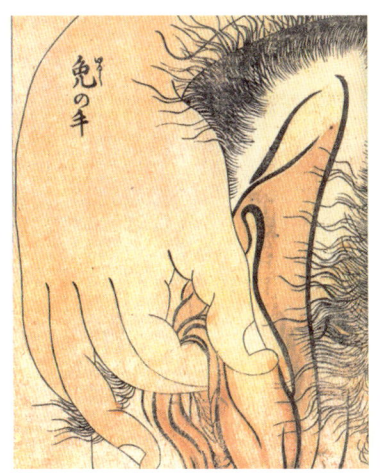 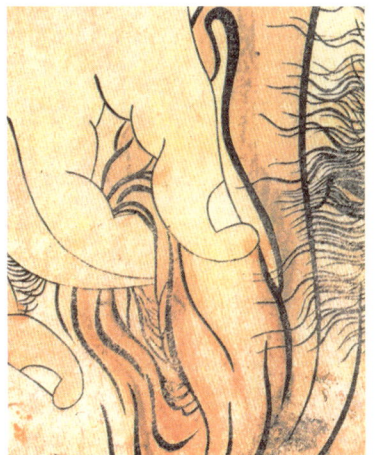

Secrets are either of the "did-you-know" or the "what-you-always-suspected" category.

Here's some "did you knows". Did you know that:

• The clitoris is not small knob at the top juncture of the inner vaginal lips, but the exterior glans of a much larger internal organ – about the same size as the male genitalia?

- The clitoral glans is packed with more sensory nerves than any other organ or site in the human body – male or female?

- The clitoris has no function except pleasure? And that...

- No other part of the human body, male or female, can make that claim?

For the purposes of this little book, we're going to note the position of the cervix, the uterus, and the ovaries *(fig.1)*, but concentrate on the erotic areas of the female genitals: the just-mentioned clitoris, the vaginal canal and the "G" spot, and the inner and outer lips of the vulva.

(1) The clitoris. Thanks to the work of medical researchers and practitioners such as Helen O'Connell as well as pioneer popular educators like Fanny Fatale, Carole Queen, and the legendary Annie Sprinkle, many people – including a sizeable number of medical doctors – now know a great deal more about the real size and shape of the clitoris than before.

As you can see, the clitoris is much larger than Terry Southern's "little marble in oil." *(fig.2)* It's proportionally the same size as the male genitalia! The "little marble in oil" is the clitoral glans.

When the clitoris is aroused, the entire clitoris is aroused. It becomes swollen, tumescent, though not to the degree that the male organ does: there are no "showers or growers" here. However the vaginal lips do become visibly engorged with blood and some clitoral glans can become very pronounced indeed.

As you can see in *(fig. 2)*, the clitoris has "legs" (crura) which extend outwards and partly explain why the inside of the female thigh is such a powerful erogenous zone. Female lubrication puzzled

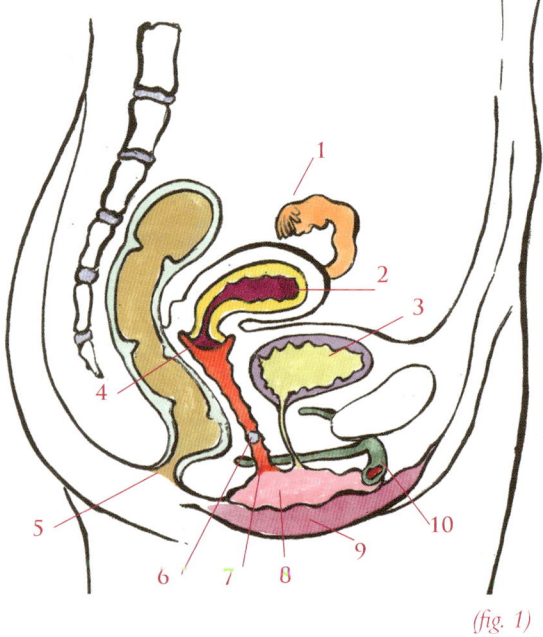

(fig. 1)

1. *Ovary*
2. *Uterus*
3. *Bladder*
4. *Cervix*
5. *Anus*
6. *G-Spot*
7. *Vagina*
8. *Inner labia*
9. *Outer labia*
10. *Clitoris*

anatomists for ages. Until a few decades ago "the glands of Bartholin," located just inside the vagina, were deemed responsible for the clear slippery liquid, analogous to male pre-ejaculate fluid, signalling sexual excitement.

We now know that sexual lubrication comes from a number of different areas, but one in particular became an object of much speculation and controversy when Dr. Ernest Grafenberg "discovered" it. This was the "G" spot.

(2) The "G" spot. Ah, the G-spot. The jackpot button. Locate it, beckon it hither, and reap its rewards. But before attempting to operate this most famous play-station, however, it would be profitable to understand a bit about its function and its relation to the rest of the female genital complex.

Despite overwhelming evidence, debate still goes on around this

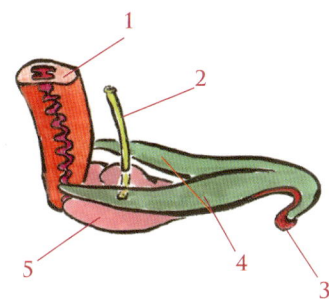

(fig. 2)

1. *Vagina*
2. *Urethra*
3. *Glans*
4. *Crura*
5. *Vestibular bulb*

organ, physically a part of the clitoris. It is now at least officially recognised as the urethral sponge, and unofficially as the location of the famed G-Spot.

The vaginal canal itself has relatively fewer nerves than the clitoris. But about one-half to two inches inside the anterior canal (that is, if the woman is lying on her back, anterior would mean at the roof of the vaginal canal), there is a spongy, ribbed mass of erectile tissue surrounding the female urethra (much like the male prostate). Proper stimulation of this area could produce both a seriously pleasurable orgasm and, with a very sizeable minority, a rush of mainly colourless, odourless, tasteless fluid.

The urethral sponge contains the para-urethral gland, which emits this ejaculate fluid through 32 tiny ducts opening into the floor of the urethra. The feeling of built-up fluid in the urethra is also akin to the feeling of needing to pee however, which can be a source of great embarrassment and anxiety for the inexperienced.

Because the ejaculate comes out of the urethra, it is commonly mistaken for urine (which comes from a different source, the bladder, which is fed from the kidneys). It is true that there is some urine detected in female ejaculate, but this varies and for the most part is undetectable.

But far from being a cause for embarrassment, female ejaculation should be taken for what it is – a very physical and thrilling manifestation of the female orgasm. And those cunnilinguists fortunate enough to find themselves on the receiving end of such an ejaculation may find it adds a new dimension to their own enjoyment of the act. Certainly there is nothing "wrong" with it, and there is nothing "wrong" if it doesn't happen, either.

Stimulation of the sponge is as

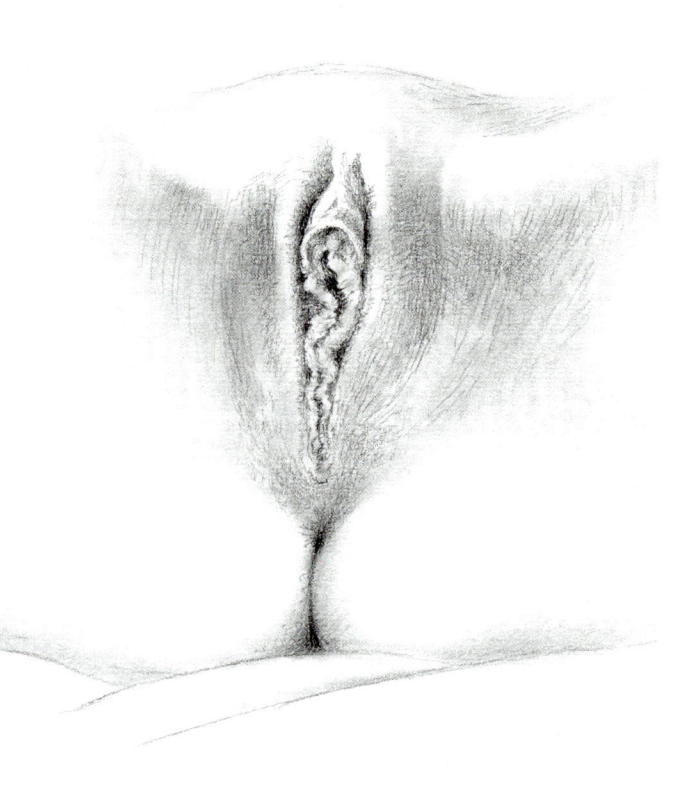

Various Types of Vulva:
This page:
Shaven
Opposite:
Black is Beautiful

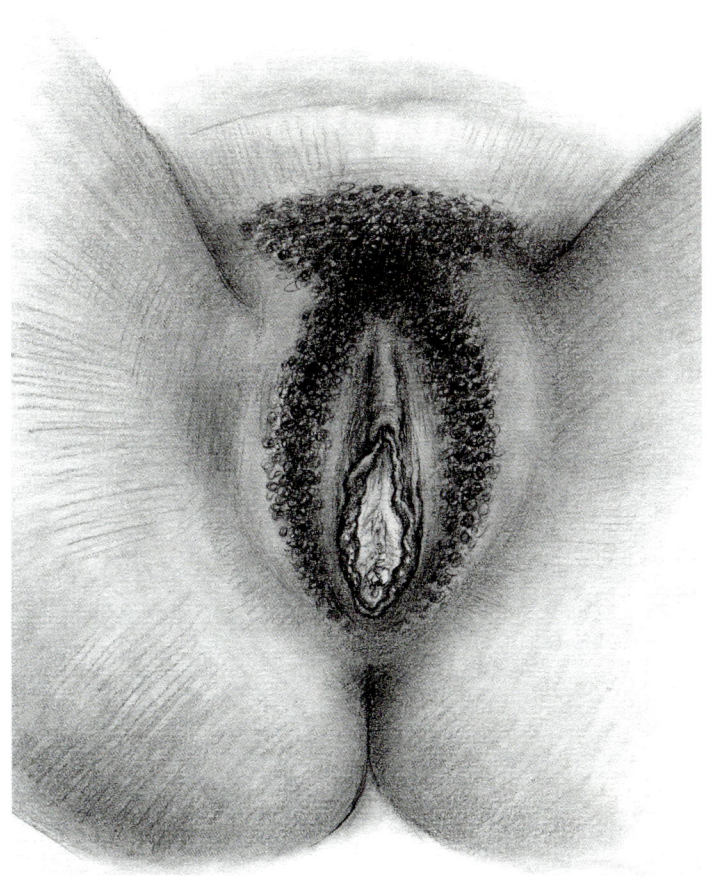

BETTER THAN TV

"It took me ages to let my inhibitions fly and have someone go down on me because I always thought my pussy looked somehow odd and I would be teased about it. The first guy who complimented me on it and told me how much he enjoyed looking at it still doesn't realise how much confidence he gave me!"

THE FIVE SENSES: SIGHT

THE VULVA — WAIT! Don't just dive in there without appreciating this wonderful part of the human body: take some time to gaze at it in all its splendour, to admire and explore at leisure. Every female has a different picture to show you: a virginal young woman with labia minora tucked away, almost out of sight; a middle-aged mother with flamboyant pussy-lips like the petals of a fleshy rose. Whether White or Afro, Asian or coffee-coloured, everyone is broadly the same but wonderfully individual. Get to recognize her different states of arousal and enjoy the show when she becomes gloriously wet and swollen, pink and suffused, like some exotic fruit. Enjoy with your eyes — but don't keep it to yourself — tell the owner what a beautiful pussy she has. And there are cosmetic changes that you can discuss - the various shaving options, for instance — or pussy jewellery, perhaps...

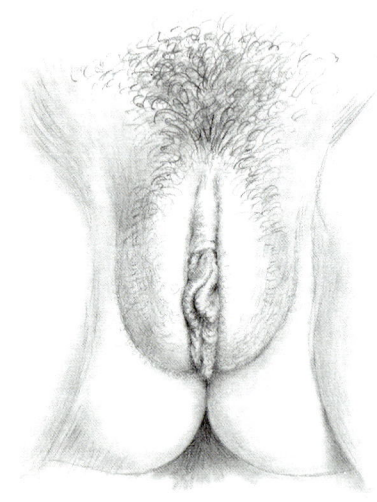

VIVE LA DIFFERENCE!

WOMEN TEND TO THINK that their vulvas might be in some way 'different' or 'wrong', their labia too 'untidy' or big. The truth is that there is no 'norm' in the detail, only in the basic anatomy. Pussy lips can be big, small, long, short, thick, thin, wide, narrow, exuberant, neat, and so on. But everyone has the external lips (labia majora), the small internal ones (labia minora) and the clitoris and its hood at the top, the urethra (pee hole) further down; below that the opening to the vagina, the perineum (the strip of skin between vagina and anus) and finally the anus at the bottom. Whatever your shape or size, you can be sure that your pussy will love being gone down on. And that's what counts...

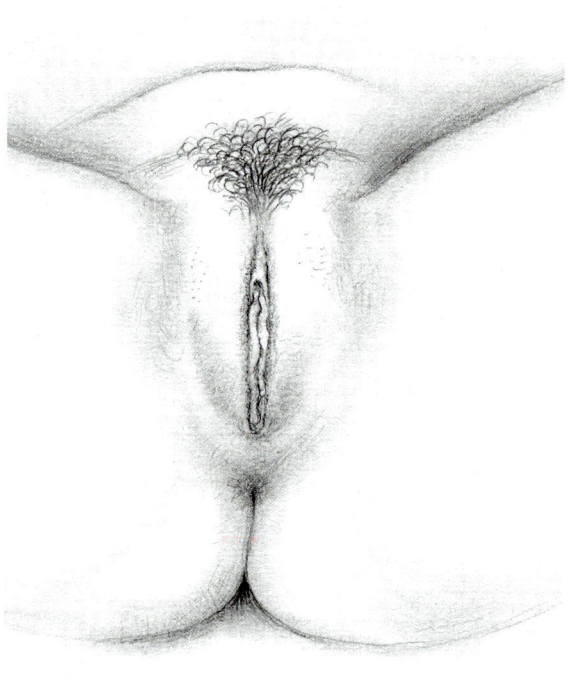

Various Types of Vulva:
This page:
Winged Lips
Opposite:
Big Outer Lips, Mature Woman; Small Neat Lips, Partially Shaven

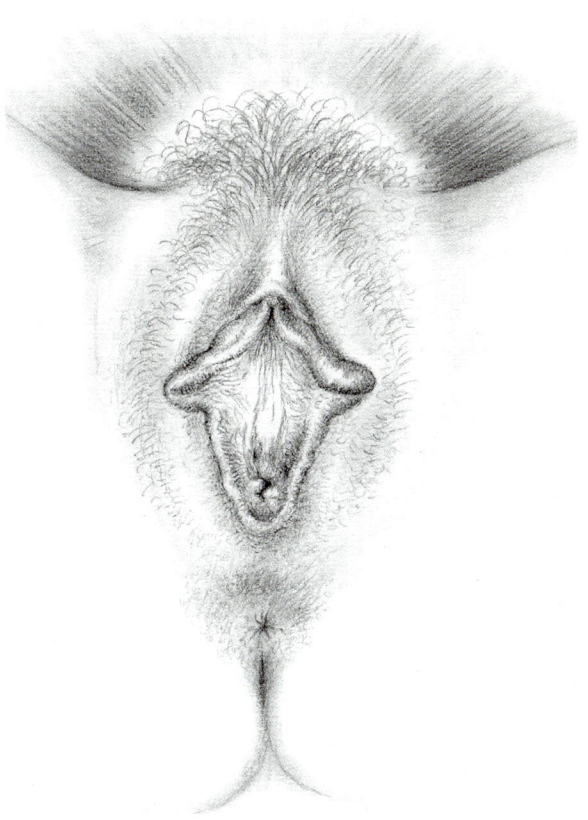

variable as stimulation of the clitoral glans. There are different spots, which respond to different kinds of stimulation at different times. We'll get to all that later, but for now, it's worth remembering that the nerve complex supporting the external clitoral glans is different from the much larger complex of nerves invigorating the urethral sponge.

(3) The Inner and Outer Lips (Labia). The inner and outer lips of the vulva cover the entrance to the vagina and urethra and are capable of arousal, and of being stimulated to arousal. They vary in size and appearance. Sometimes the inner lips protrude outside the outer lips, and this as well as other media-induced anxieties about genital appearance has given rise to a growing branch of cosmetic surgery. It's as well to remember that beauty is very much in the eye of the beholder, and that really most of us do not subscribe to a standard aesthetic when it comes to genitalia, female – or male for that matter.

One of the funniest and saddest stories about the appearance of human female genitals has now left our solar system. The space-probe Pioneer II, now well past the orbit of Pluto, contains a metal disc, crammed with information about our world. It also features a line drawing of a male and female human being.

The figures are racially indeterminate; political correctness has been observed. One small anatomical detail is missing, however. Although the male has a penis and, if the aliens understand perspective, two testicles, the female has no vaginal lips at all. Where her vulva should be, there is only a blank "V."

Be they insectoid, gas, liquid, or flying amoebas, whatever kind of intelligent life form in the cosmos discovers this small football-sized encyclopedia, it will forever be puzzled as to the reproductive anatomy of one-half of the human

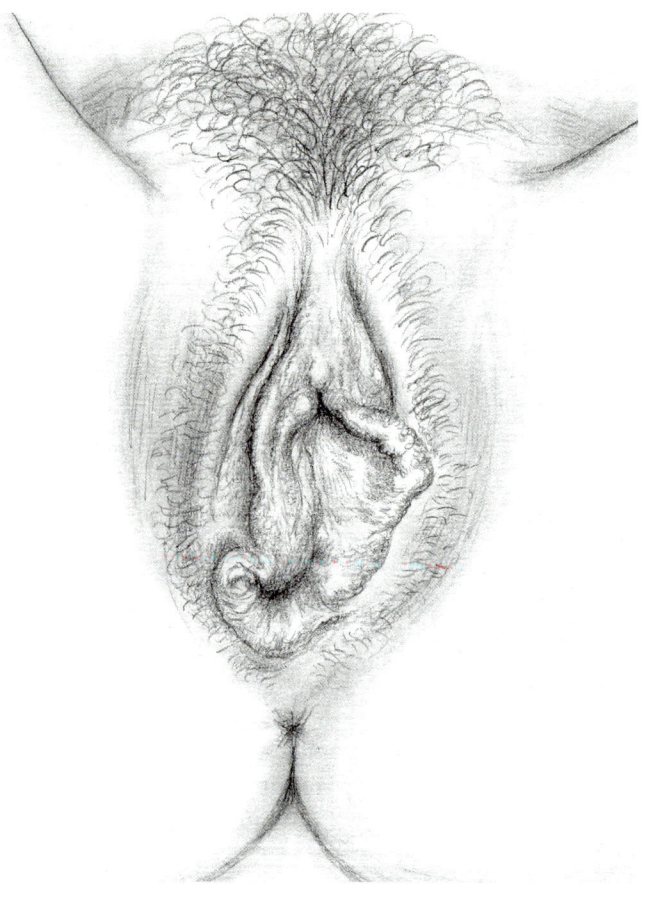

Various Types of Vulva:
This page: **Big, Exuberant Lips**
Opposite: **Gloriously Hairy**

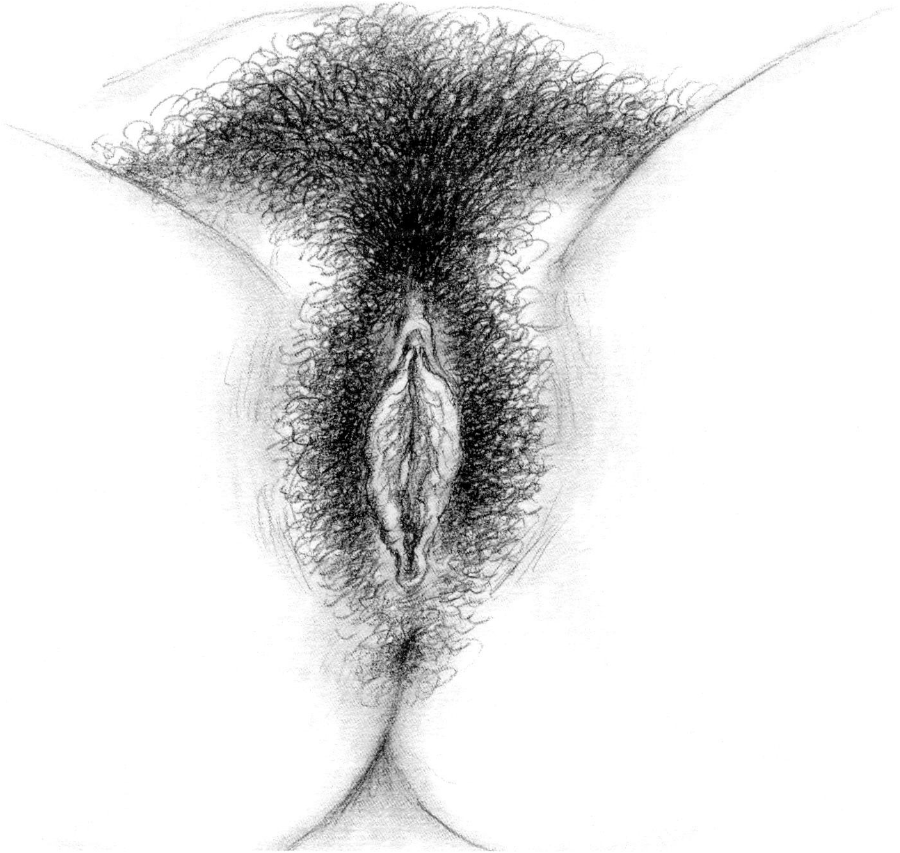

species. Evidence of our shame and fear is now speeding through the infinite reaches of space for eternity.

So let's concentrate on what's really important. We've looked briefly at the anatomy of the female sexual parts. Now let's look at some of the ways we can give them pleasure.

DON'T BE SHY

TELL HIM YOU WANT TO BE EATEN! Sometimes lovers miss out on cunnilingus because it hasn't arisen in conversation about what we like best. Sometimes the woman is simply too inhibited to ask for it. Most lovers will suggest it as a matter of course - or just do it without asking as a natural part of foreplay. But if they haven't and you are too shy to ask - don't be. If your lover is worth his salt he'll respond enthusiastically and sensitively. But help him by telling him what you like and guiding him if he gets it wrong.

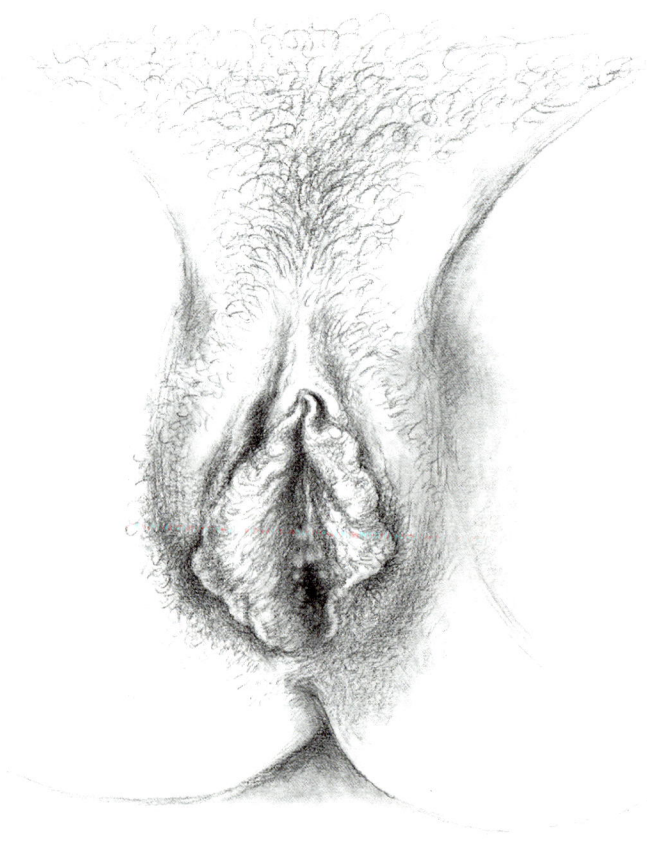

Various Types of Vulva
This page:
Mature, Post-childbirth, Luscious

II WHY SEX TIPS
DO NOT (ALWAYS) HELP

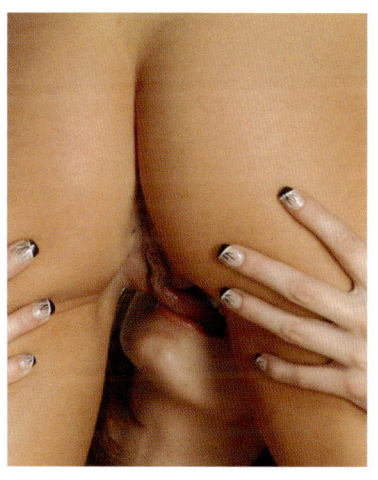
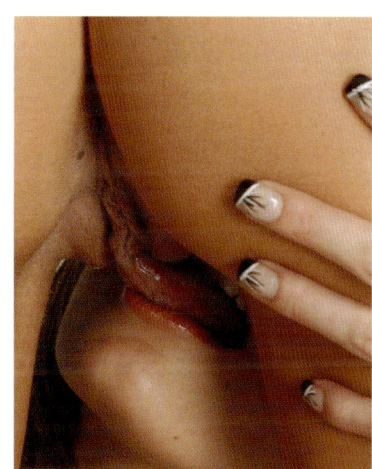

"She had this bored look on her face the whole time," he said.
"What were you doing?" I asked.
"The alphabet thing, like in the magazine article."
"The alphabet thing – ?"
"You know, where you 'write' the alphabet around the clit with your tongue? I wrote the whole alphabet. Nothing. I even wrote sexy words. Nothing."
"You mean she just lay there?"

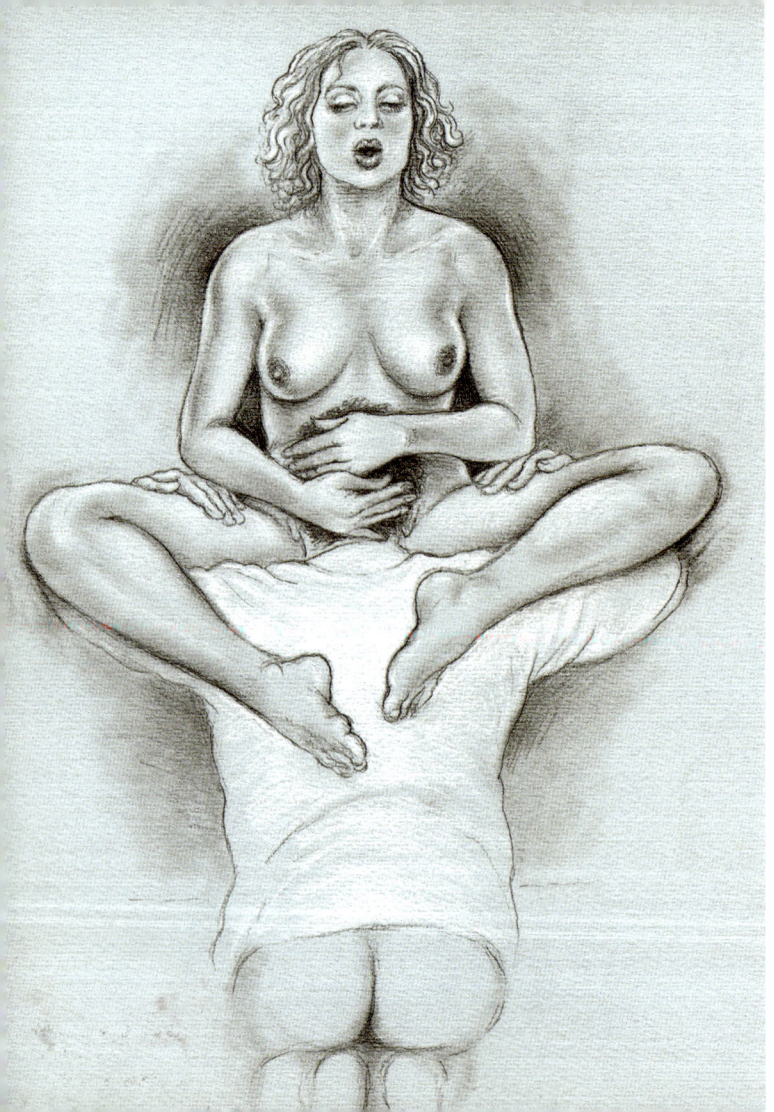

FEAR NOT...

"I was worried about what it would be like when I first dived down there. Sex had always been quite sticky and messy, with some fairly exotic odours, so I naturally assumed that it would be the same when I went down on her. But it was alright, because the pheromones kicked in and suddenly it was the best sort of intimate messiness and she tasted great - the smells were good, too."

Hands On
Communicate with your hands on the back of your lover's head if they can't see you. It can give you (the receiver) a delicious sense of control and authority.

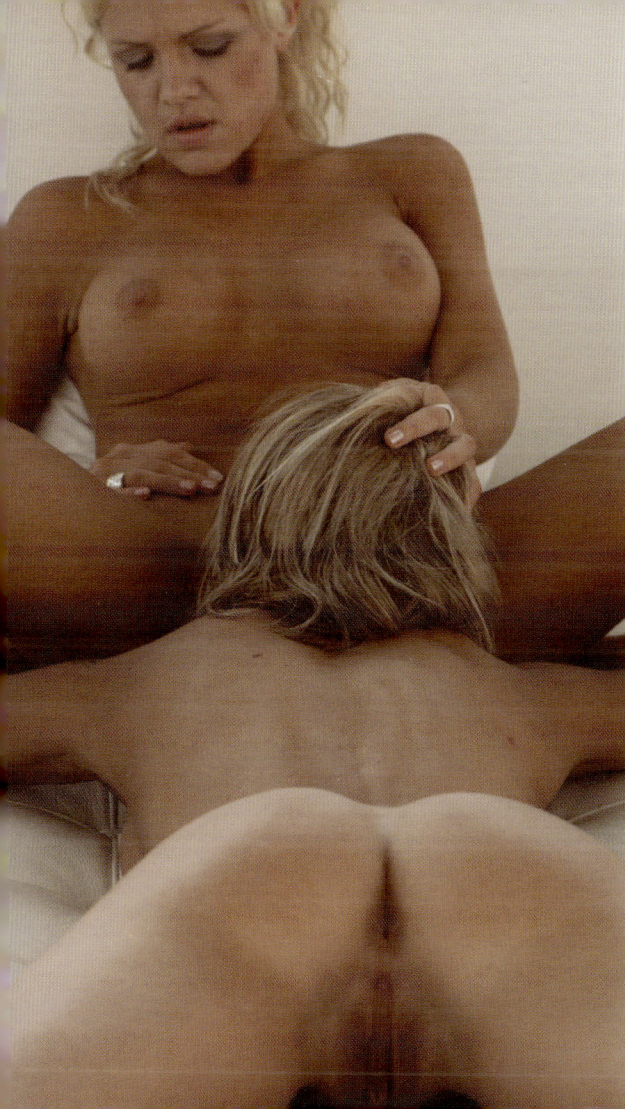

"Well, she did correct my spelling once or twice…"

If physical technique was all there was to it, the number of "sex-tips" in magazine articles, books, sex-help websites, and the rest would have given us all mastery of the Art of Cunnilingus. Alas, not so.

The best response any of us can make to the difference between the promise offered by "Sex-Tips" articles and our own experience is that we are "learning."

But what exactly are we learning? Cunnilingus with ice-cubes? Mints? Strawberries? Under the table in a restaurant? Figure eights with the tongue? Algebraic symbols? Lapping it like a dog? Doggie-style? Or soixante-neuf?

And then there are the myriad

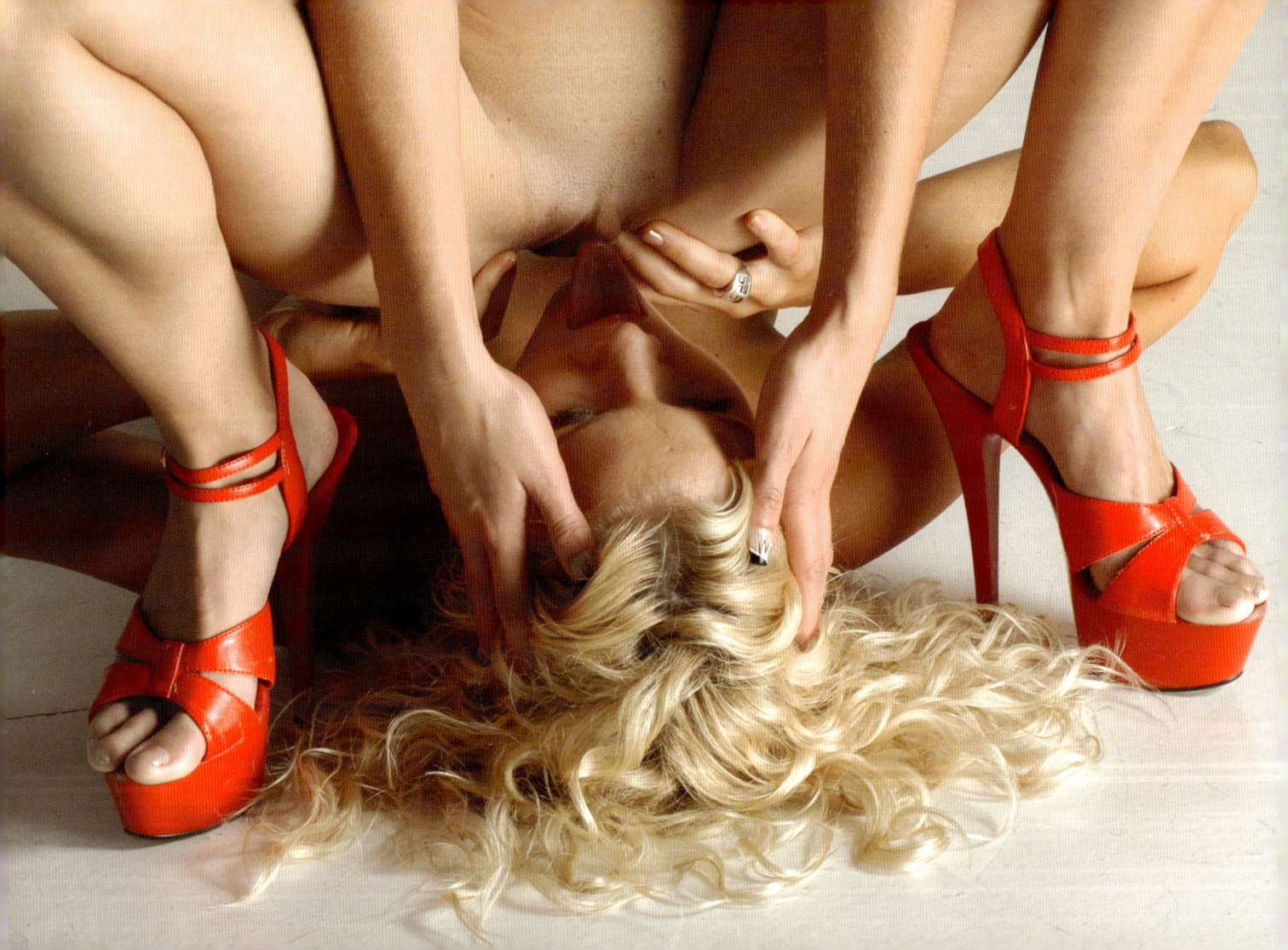

ways of mouth-to-genital-congress developed by thousand-year-old cultures with poetic names for each technique like "Hummingbird Sipping Nectar."

So much to learn, so little time…

Oh, and don't you just love all those personal anecdotes in the boxes we see on the side of sex "How-To" books, like, "…but when I did "X" she tore the pillow in half and screamed words in a foreign language neither of us knew. It's been bliss ever since."

I don't know about you, but all I want to do is hit that blissful couple with a rolled-up newspaper. When you try "X" and the only response is a diplomatic shift in position, it does not mean you're "no good." No: sex tips alone are no guarantee of anything, and running through

THE FIVE SENSES: TOUCH

THE VAGINAL AREA is a playground for the senses and touch is no exception: the variety of skin textures is sheer delight for sensitive tongues, lips or fingertips. From rough to smooth, from the labia's wrinkly exterior to the slick membraneous interior, even the surrounding hair can differ in feel (although a pubic hair in the mouth can be infuriatingly distracting and is best removed forthwith).

Letting your tongue stay dry until it can sense the arrival of lubrication, too, is a magical moment. Try finding the urethra with the very tip of your tongue. Feeling the labia becoming fuller, less pliable and 'floppy', more turgid and sensing the same thing with the clitoris is another brilliant sensation. Though not strictly-speaking cunnilingus, why not use the sensitive tip of your nose, too?

one after another is no proof of expertise.

So how do you find what works for both of you, before desperation or boredom ruins the whole idea? Without feeling self-conscious, without ruing spontaneity, and just plain sexual ecstasy?

Fortunately, there is a simple approach that will allow you to move easily from one technique to another, be it Tantric, New Age, or Boogie; an approach which may help to make each encounter an experience of effortless discovery and invention!

I call it "Tongue Talking."

Before we get into that, it must be noted that the Art Of Cunnilingus, despite the dictionary definition, is not just confined to the tongue.

Or the mouth. Or even (a general favourite) the fingers and mouth and tongue. Like everything else, Art begins with Attitude. Attitude defines Approach.

Even the most inarticulate 20-something football star will try his utmost to explain that great playing is not just a question of bashing the ball in the general direction of the goal. He will try to tell you no two teams are the same; no two games are the same. You have to know your opponent; you have to assess the situation. Technique by itself won't score.

And so it is with sex, and particularly cunnilingus. Who are you with? What does she want? What does she like, and when? And the last, but by no means the least of the great five "W's," why are you doing what you're doing?

As an old time popular entertainer's tag line went, "I wanna tell you a story." Everybody likes a good story.

What makes a good story? The elements are simple. First, you Set The Scene. The great writer Elmore Leonard advises, "Never start out with the weather. Start with the person." How true. Whether you're in a one-night stand or a long-term relationship, you start with whom you're with, and make sure they know you know.

The next element of a good story is the Proposition. Here, you don't have to worry about inspiration: the proposition is Your Mouth On Her Vulva – and what will happen next. The suspense is built in.

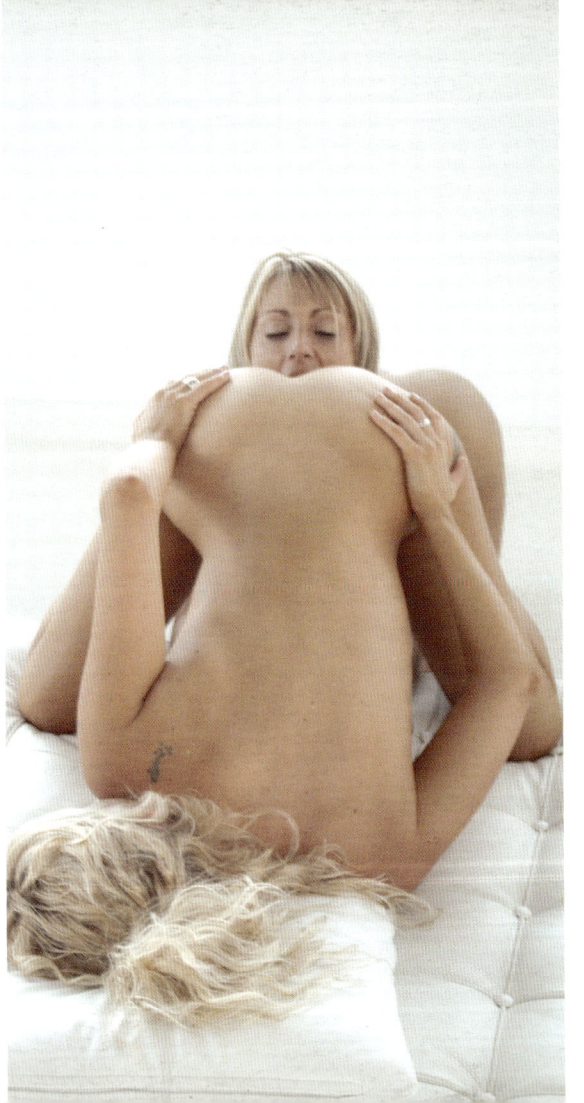

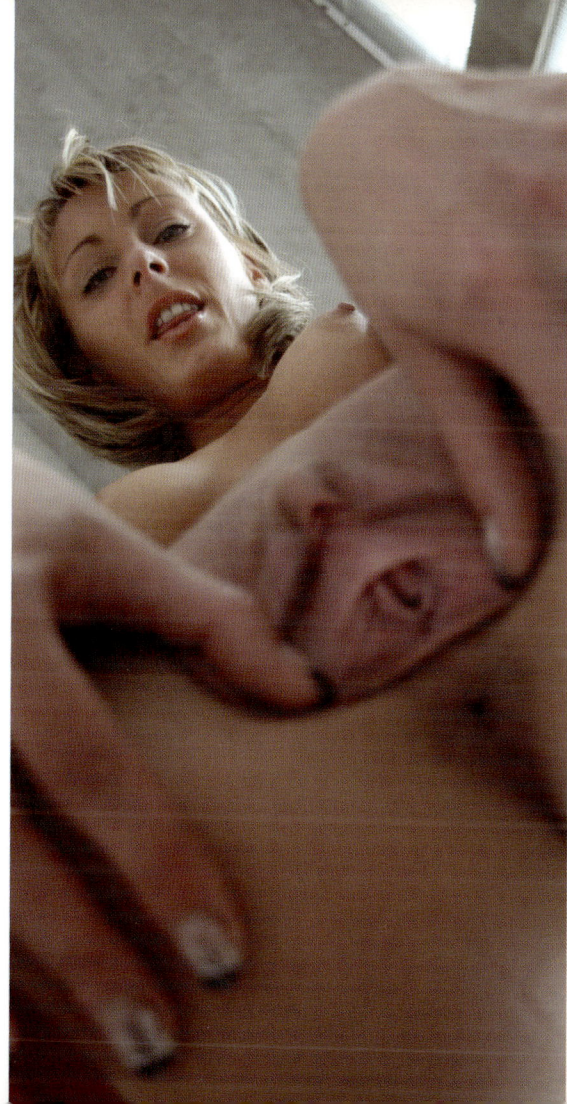

CHECK OUT YOUR PERSONAL EQUIPMENT: TONGUE

SOME CLASSIC MOVES for an agile tongue. These include writing the alphabet (corny but fun); slow, relaxed circles around the clitoris – trace your tongue around the hood without touching the clit itself; rapid, short, upward licks punctuated by little 'stabs' into the vaginal tunnel; side to side, then up and down; with the tip of your tongue, trace a path down the valleys and over the ridges of both sets of labia, increasing the pressure as you go; make your tongue flat and broad as if you were licking ice cream, if met with approval, keep the pressure firm; keep alternating all of the above until she finds one she loves. Your tongue will probably be the first victim of a marathon muffing – it will tire. So if it does, give it a rest and just think of it as training fatigue – you'll go for longer next time.

The third element is Development. Let me repeat that: Development. This means not giving the plot away by going straight to the clitoral glans and tonguing and sucking – it's not the final scene yet! It is here you begin to employ different techniques, all of which should fit the context of what you're doing.

All good stories develop using surprise, suspense, and diversion. But the "story" you're telling depends on your response to the way your "listener" (your partner, that is) guides your inspiration.

For example, if she immediately grabs you by the ears and attempts to pull your head into her womb, while making noises you only hear on wildlife recordings, your approach and subsequent "story" will of course be different from the vocabulary you employ if the minute your lips make contact she flings out her arms limply and sighs as if floating away on a peaceful cloud.

What that is, is up to you both, but usually, generally, the end of cunnilingus means the beginning of something else. However the best stories never let you forget the importance of the climax to the characters themselves.

How do you register this? Eye contact, talking to each other, or, if the position (such as sixty-nine) limits that, by the way your hands express your appreciation.

Now let's look at some of those story-telling techniques.

CHECK OUT YOUR PERSONAL EQUIPMENT: TONGUE (contd.)

THINK OF YOUR TONGUE as another finger, but one that comes with its own lubrication, is infinitely variable in its texture and firmness and incredibly sensitive. And it can taste, too, which is more than your fingers can do. The tongue is a wonderfully powerful muscle that can vary its texture by relaxing or tensing. It can go into a phallic point, it can become floppy and soft, it can be sinuous and sexy. Keep trying all the various permutations.

NEXT TO GODLINESS

HARRY: "We always seem to have sex in the morning, for some reason; Jillian's quite a fastidious person, and I'm always aware of this, when I go down on her, so I make sure that I've shaved (no morning beard rash, please) and we both brush our teeth. This seems to work for both of us. Obviously my mouth is fresher and more 'awake' and when we kiss orally, as well as genitally, it makes a real difference."

JILLIAN: "I feel happier when Harry has done his morning 'ablutions': although I'm not quite as fussy as he makes out, it's definitely a more pleasant experience - and who needs all that not-so-friendly bacteria. We're told that the vagina is a self-cleaning organ; so is the mouth but we're not always shoving food into our pussies!"

III STORYTELLING
TECHNIQUES: THE OPENING SCENE

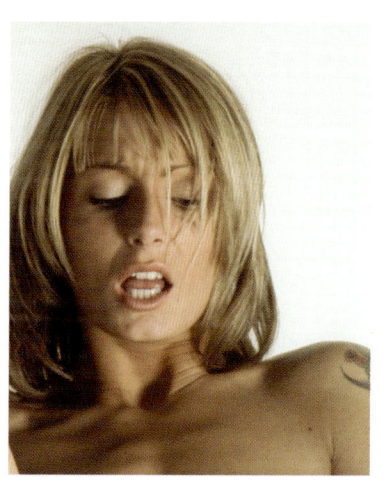 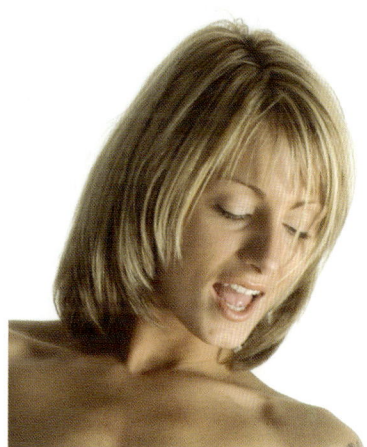

Everyone know a good storyteller when they see and hear one. The best storytellers are a bit like actors as they tell their stories.

Of course you shouldn't 'act'. But you can express your involvement to your partner; she should know you're involved. The British are not as deadpan as they make out to be. Like when they play air guitar or dance sexily in a club, or scream at the television. Plenty of faces made there!

So: release your face in the sack. Allow yourself more expression than one woman's recently dumped poker-faced partner, who was trying to get her aroused by " …just …twiddling knobs, like, you know, 'come in, Tokyo?'"

Space doesn't allow for more than one or two scenarios as an example, so however you get to these and others; whether you drop to your knees as she sits on the couch, or the kissing and fondling in bed finds you between her legs, the first thing you do is:

Appreciate what's before you.
(You can get as close as you like.)
You might even express your appreciation (optional).
But no touching it, yet.

It's a bit like looking at the titles of a hit movie you've been looking forward to seeing.

Try eye contact whenever possible

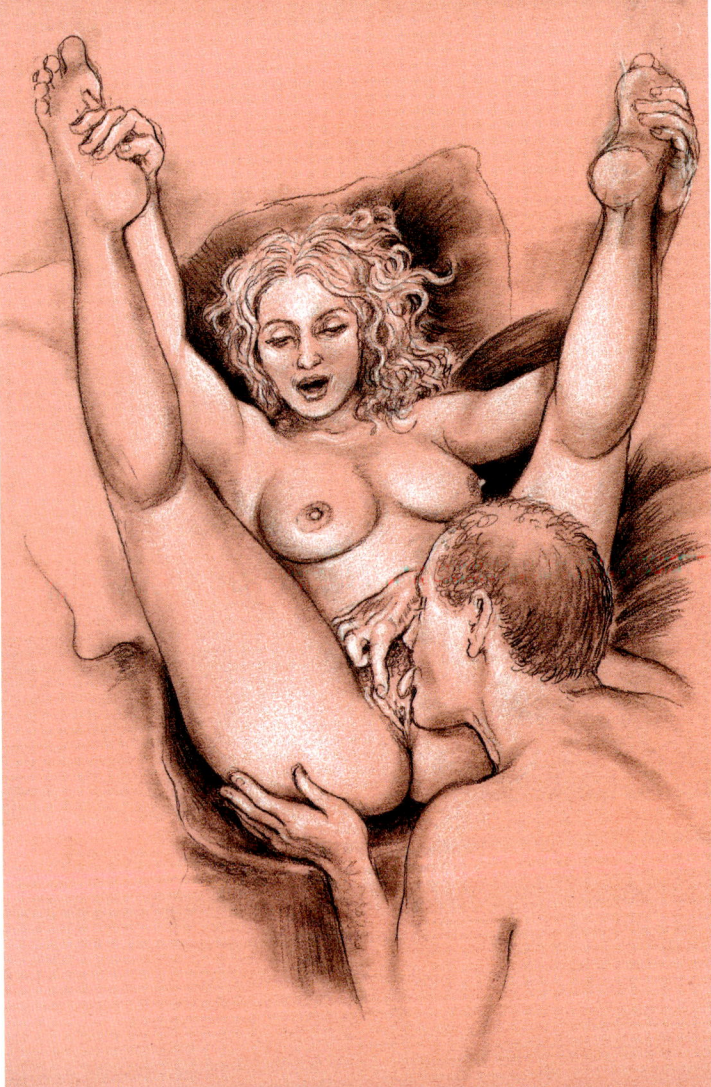

This page and opposite:
Cupping Her Buttocks to Bring Her Vulva to Your Mouth

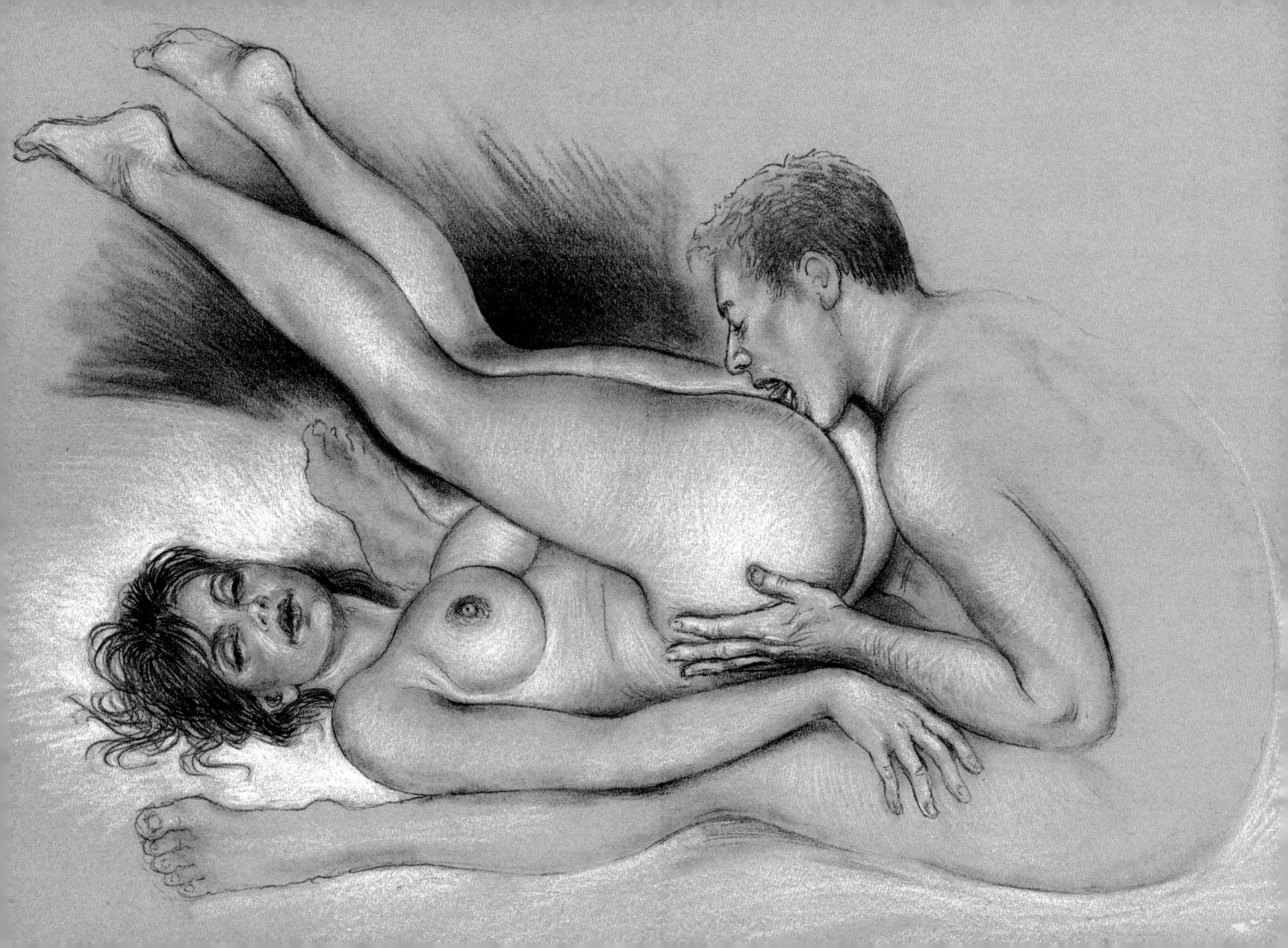

(generally very desirable). Then, whatever position you find yourself in, simply cup one hand around each buttock as you bring your mouth to her vulva or lift her vulva to your mouth.

This "opening move", or opening scene, can now progress anywhere, and in any style. Her are two basic possible (and opposite) ways to look at it:

Tantric, or New Age. In this kind of "story" you see her vulva and its inner sanctum full of cosmic potential, a special basket or vessel, brimming with transcendental mysteries, to be gradually revealed by your mouth as it closes on its rim. Eye contact here is about love and fusion of souls. Have plenty of candles around for that low-light night effect.

"Down-and-dirty" Sex. Here, as you lift her boldly, shamelessly to your mouth, you express appreciative lust. She in turn

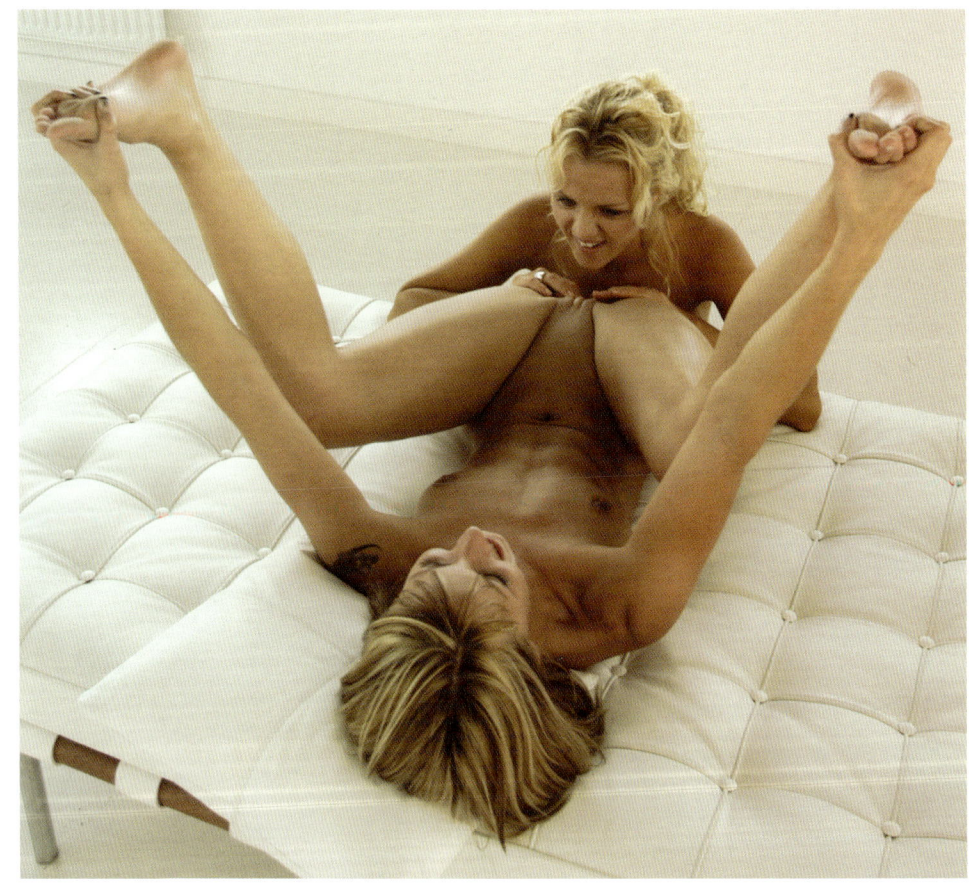

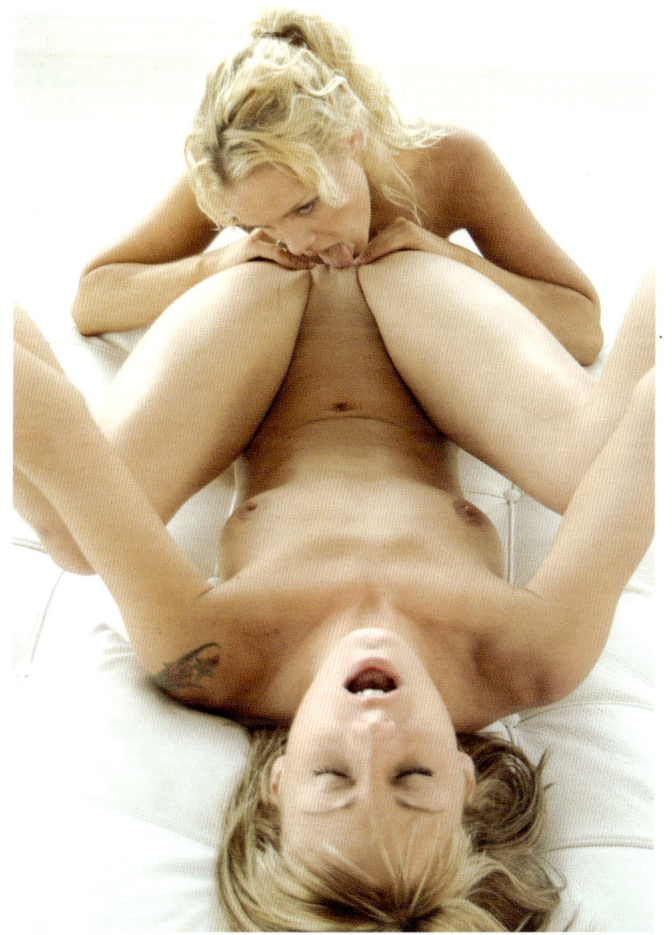

exposes her cunt for you to lick it, suck it, play with it, in order for you to give her the most intense feeling of pleasure possible from this most intimate act. Eye contact here is about conflict, the "sexual battle". Devices, lube and towels are boldly exhibited as in, "This is what's in store for you, you horny bitch!"

And – in your own time and judgement – you can switch between the two. No one will call you a dilettante.

Holding up one half of a woman's body by the buttocks can be tiring, even if she helps by arching up and bracing herself with her heels. You don't have to maintain this unless you're into body building, so after the initial impression has been established, you can ease her down and get into a more comfortable position for you both.

Remember: these are only suggestions. Suggestions which

point to a way of thinking about oral sex which uses your imagination, as well as a receptive attitude to the responses of your partner.

Remember: the listener is as important as the storyteller. (In the course of things the "listener" could easily become the "storyteller!")

MADONNA-WHORE

"When I open myself up to Frank it's a feeling of complete abandonment. I know he's looking at me, drinking it all in visually, then... literally! It's a huge turn-on to know that I turn HIM on by having me look at my pussy and I feel pleasantly sluttish, especially when I hold my legs wide apart for him. But at other times I feel like an imperious queen, directing him to lick me this way or that. Oh dear, it's kind of schizoid, I know..."

THE FIVE SENSES: TASTE

IT'S NOT FOR NOTHING that slang for cunnilingus often refers to 'eating' or 'dining'. Taste is an important part of the whole delicious experience. There are times during a woman's ovulation cycle when her 'juices' will taste different. Not more or less pleasant, just different. Diet can have an effect on the flavour of vaginal secretions too and sometimes this needs to be adjusted (hold the garlic, hold the asparagus) for 'flavour control' if the taste becomes less enjoyable. In the context, with pheromones flying wild, a whole range of flavours will be more than acceptable to the cunnilinguist. But if there's a sharp difference in taste, there could be a health issue involved, so point this out, tactfully, to your partner.

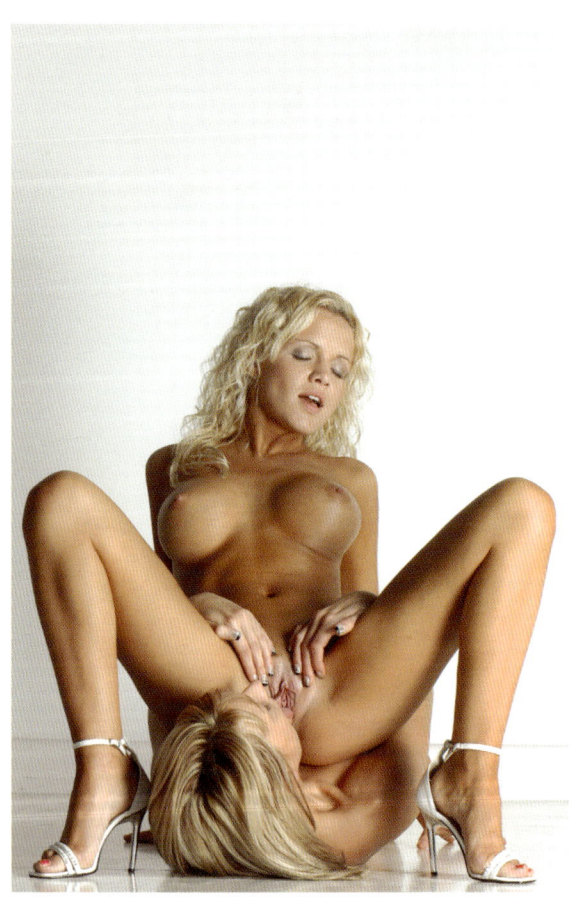

IV STORYTELLING:
THE STORY CONTINUES

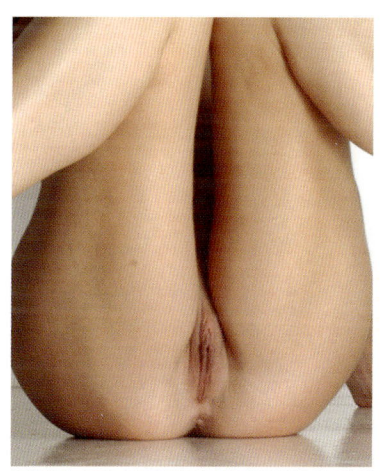 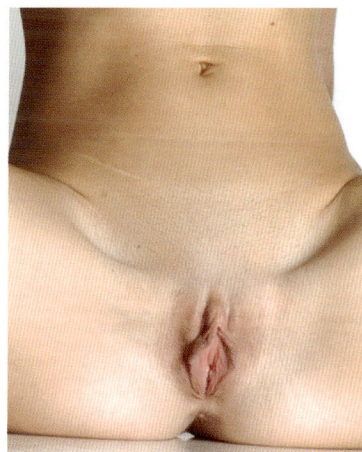

Now that your story is ready for development, here are some ideas you can build on:

The Cat
Ever see a cat play ever so gently with something? It reaches out, and strokes it delicately, delicately. There are claws in the paw, but it never uses them, and that's the thrill – you have it in your power to plunge your tongue in and give her a damn good suck, but you don't.

You explore her all over with the delicate tip of your tongue.

The Blind Tongue
If that doesn't appeal as an image, try imagining your tongue is the only thing you have to find out what her vulva looks like. It delicately traces the outlines of the outer and inner lips, above, below and around the glans – you get the idea.

The Koi Kiss
Or you can develop the scene in a secluded garden in Imperial Japan. In the middle of the garden is a pond in which large Koi swim lazily around. They are very tame, very intelligent fish, and the larger they are, the older they are and the more costly they are. If you dip the tip of your finger into the pond the Koi gently comes up to it and makes a "wow" on it with its lips (as you might go "wow" around the clitoral hood without touching the glans itself) and then smoothly glides away.

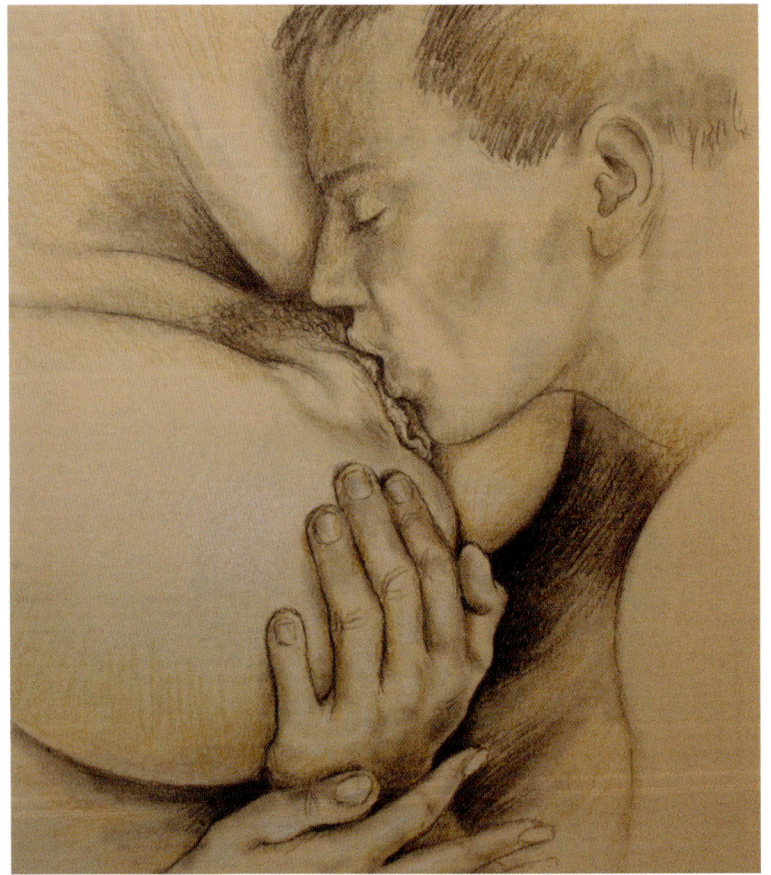

The 'Surprised by Koi' Kiss

The 'Turtle'

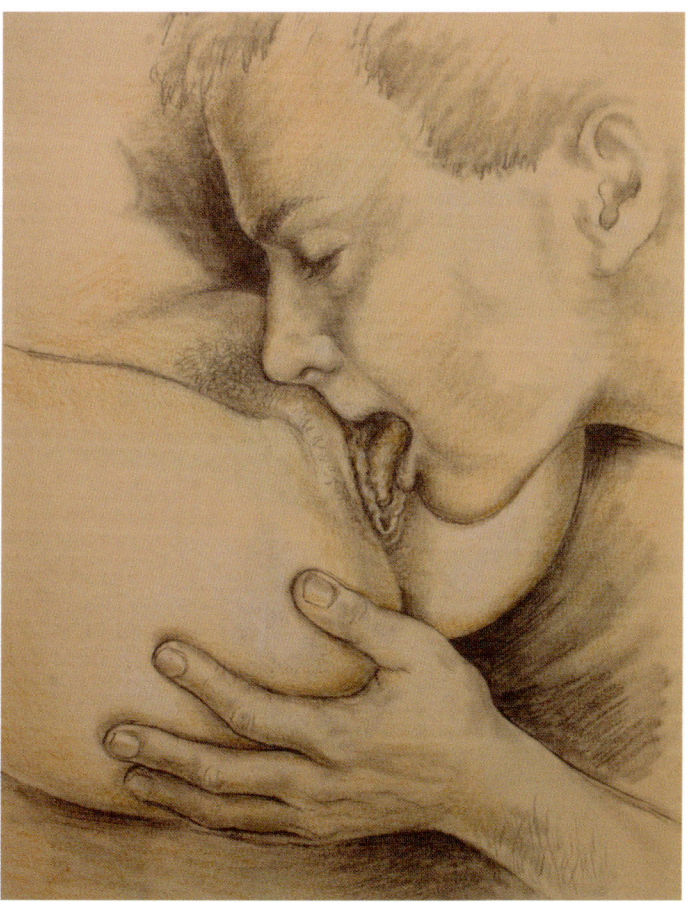

The Turtle

FADE IN: A tropical, deserted sandy beach. There's no one for miles. It's where the giant sea turtles hang out. You can see one, down the beach. It gives you an idea. Your top lip comes down to cover the teeth (we don't want that "ouch!" at all, ever) and anchors itself above the clitoral hood.

In a way, your upper jaw looks a bit like a turtle's top beak, leaving your lower lip and tongue free to probe the entrance of the vagina, or to gently lick or apply pressure to the area just under the clitoral glans.

You can vary this module by moving your head rapidly up and down, your top lip (covering the teeth!) hitting above the clitoral glans again in imitation of the heterosexual penetrative act.

Tongue-Fuck
This is where the tongue is extended as long and as stiff as possible, and

thrusts, with long strokes, in and out of the vagina (keeping the lips well over the teeth) in imitation of an erect phallus. It is both faintly ridiculous and, for the receptive mind, intensely naughty.

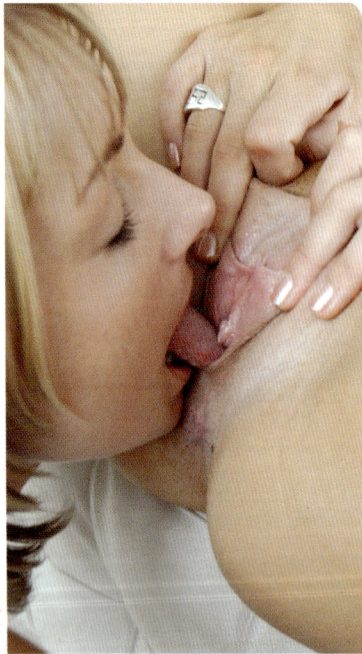

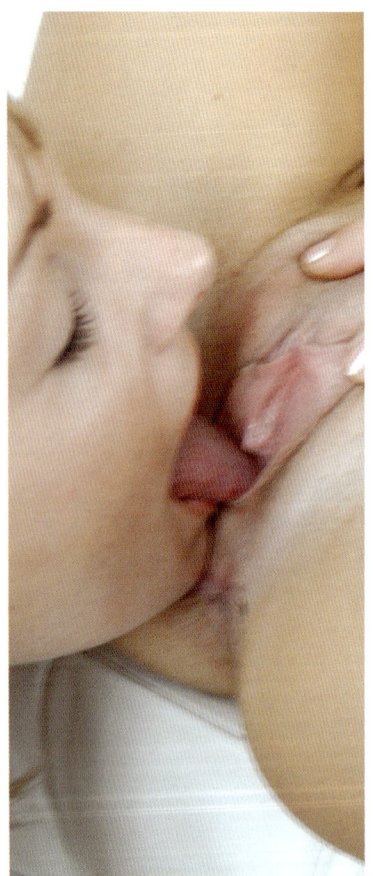

Sub-Plot
Now leave the area with a lick and a promise and, with your mouth and tongue (no teeth!) give the insides of her legs, from the vulva to about halfway down the thigh, a good, sexy mouth massage. It's good if you close on the area just outside the vulva: there are a few good nerves there which could use it.

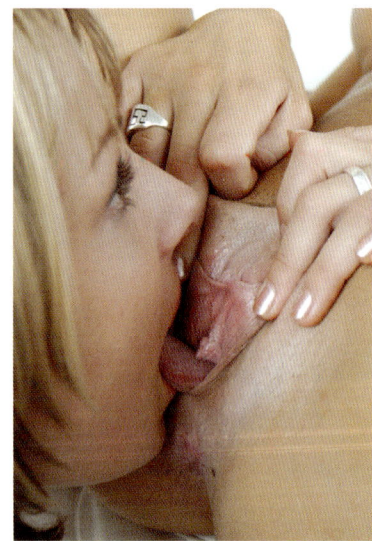

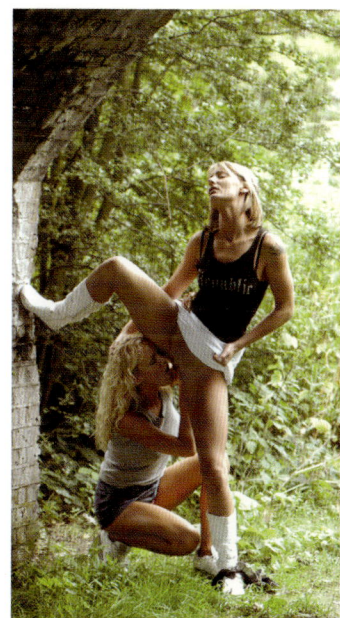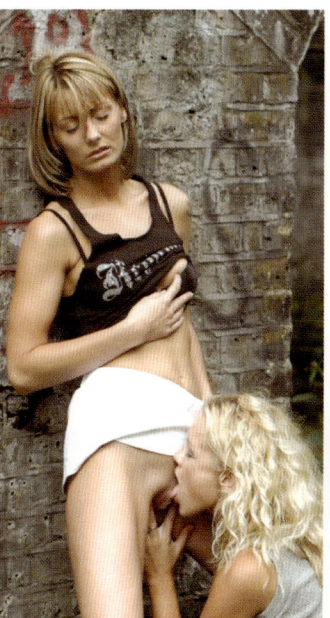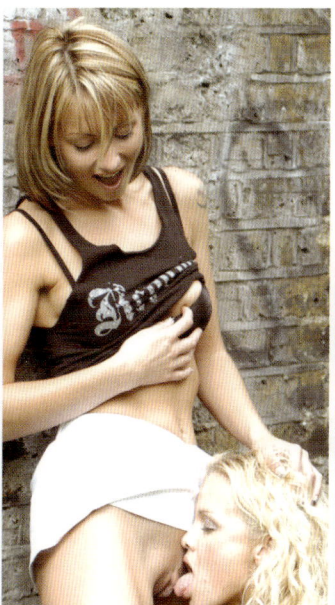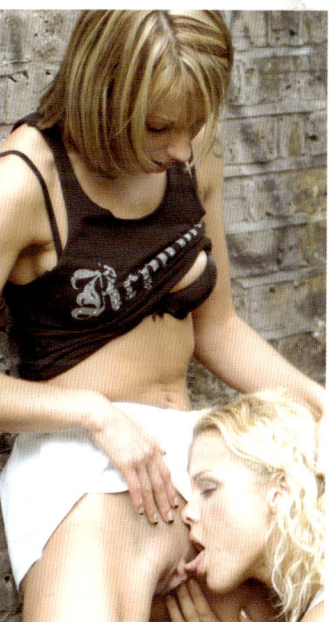

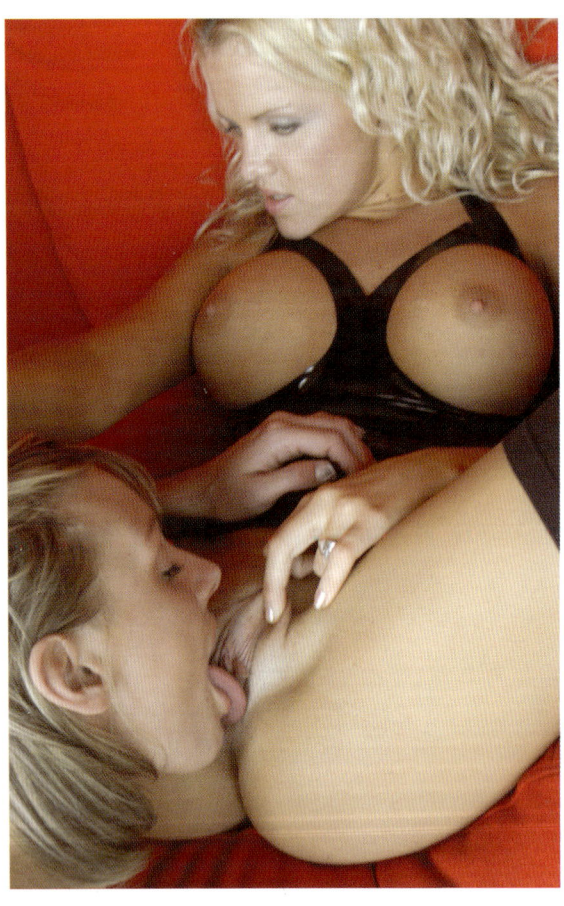

The First Kiss
The plot thickens, as should the labial lips. Again, making sure the teeth are covered by your lips, gently pull and suck on the labia majora, and the labia minora, too.

Lap-Dog
I recommend saving this for the end of your opening chapter, although you can return to it any time, and again. It's so "out there," so "in your face," so to speak, that I think it best it's used sparingly: Lap all of her vulva, her vaginal opening, like a dog, with your tongue as wide and as flat as possible.

There. Think about these images, think of others. You don't have to go through the alphabet, yet. You don't have to make that rapid lizard tongue-flicking of the adolescent rock n' roll musician – yet. You don't even have to make humming noises with your nose pressed against her pubic bone like a demented electric shaver, yet. And you haven't even touched the clitoral glans – yet.

Stimulation of the inside of the thigh next to the vulva with the mouth without touching the vulva itself can provide intense pleasure and even orgasm, but would take a great deal of room to describe adequately.

With just these few modules in play you will establish yourself as a cunnilingual sophisticate, a tongue-talker, beginning the kind of tale the receiving partner cannot help but think, "Hmmm, tell me more…"

ATHLETIC SPRINTING

"I went jogging with a girl I really fancied and we'd just got back to my place when she complained about being really stiff: 'Can you just give my calves a quick rub?' turned into a fully-fledged, legs-behind-ears tongue-fucking event. She came about three times and then she sucked me to a fantastic climax. It was the best oral sex I ever had..."

V HAND POSITIONS
AND DEVICES

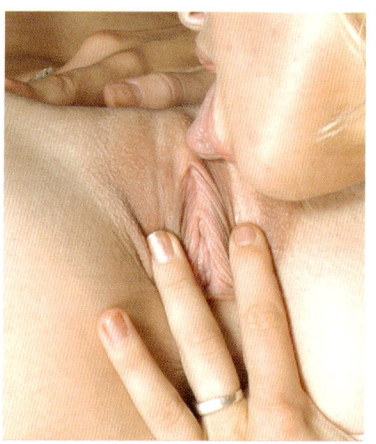 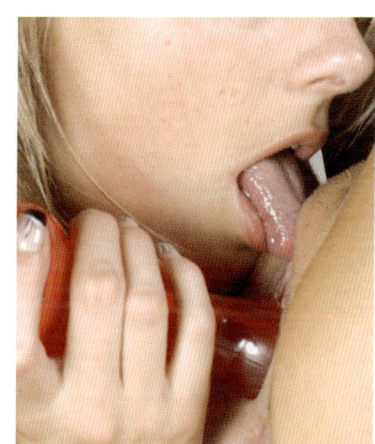

We've now explored the extraordinary anatomy of the female genitalia and some neighbouring erogenous zones. We've looked at the concept of "Tongue Talking," a way of using ideas and images to "tell" a kind of "story," using your mouth and hands and tongue.

The concept of "Tongue Talking" allows you to incorporate all the tips and tricks you can find in most magazines and books – without making them feel like tips and tricks from most magazines and books..

So far we've only opened the "story", appreciated the "opening scene" and looked at ways to "develop" it. So far we haven't touched the clitoral glans, or done anything more energetic than prepare for "plot complications", like surprise, suspense, and diversion.

I can assure the impatient that some techniques will be discussed here and in the following chapters. But let's not lose the plot now. You've introduced the story; the proposition is set; you've developed it; and now you're into the climax, the chase, the denouement, the final part, in which everything is made clear and no questions or surprises remain.

It's now time to consider the use of your hands, positions, and devices, as well as your mouth and tongue to develop your "story". They are,

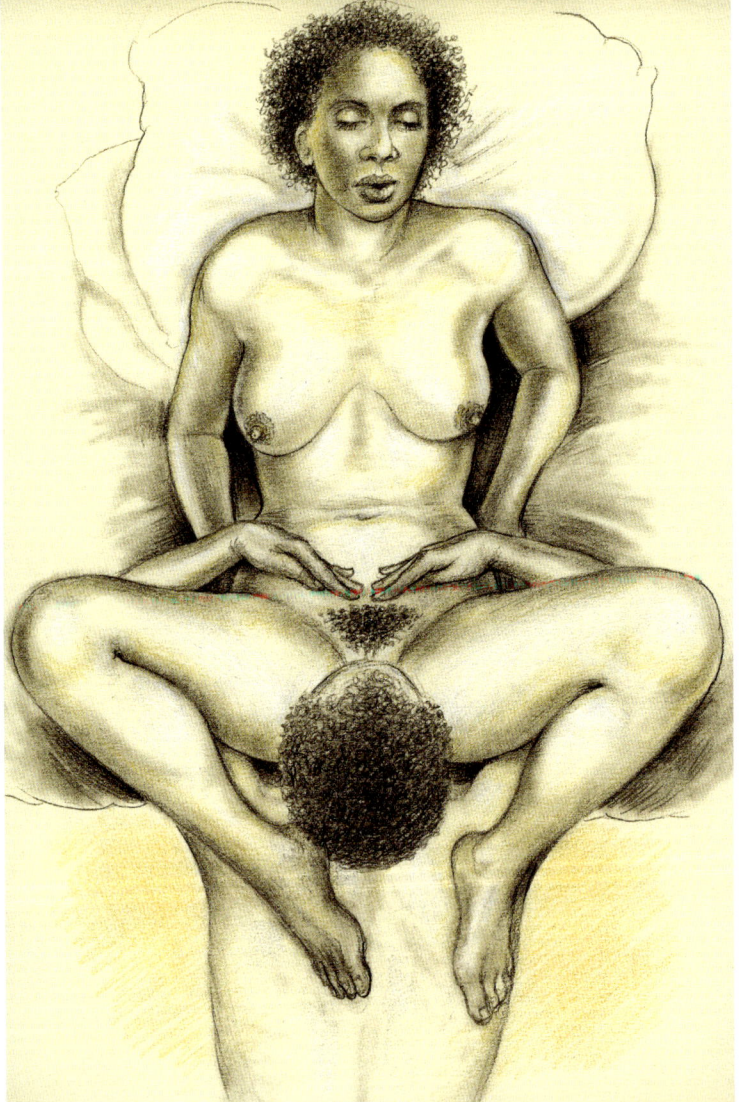

The 'M' Frame

of course, essential in developing the situation (although devices are "extras" by definition).

Oh, And By the Way
In this situation, hands mean clean hands. Your hands should be as well tended as a violinist's and as safe as a doctor's.

Questionable cleanliness will always produce hesitation in your partner, and an 'ouch!' reaction always knocks the sexual temperature down a few notches, not to say a major distraction from plot-interest.

Basic Positions
A look at some basic opening hand positions will no doubt inspire the beginning or advanced cunning linguist to explore or develop his or her own original variations.

Your hands can be positioned in various ways, whether you've surprised her in the kitchen, joined her in the shower, approached her on the couch, or kneeling on front of her as she stands on the bed.

But soon you will generally both be lying down, and here is where basic body positions come into play. In both of the positions I'm about to describe, she is on her back.

The "M"
Begin with this simplest: it will allow both parties to warm-up. Her thighs rest either on your shoulders or your neck. Your face is up against her vulva. Your arms now encircle her thighs and your hands meet naturally on her mons pubis, the area covered by most thongs.

Your thumbs should now be pointing inward and down; your first finger tips should be able to touch. The shape your hands are making are a bit like the letter "M." This is also the best position to hum while you work.

This position has the added advantage of being able to apply gentle pressure just above her pubic bone with the outside fingers, and aside from this stimulation it can give to some of the muscles involved in orgasm, it also give the impression that you are "in charge", which many women find extra-pleasurable.

The first position allows for a more romantic, "unthreatening" beginning; you can use this first position for your entire "story", if you wish.

An alternate beginning position depends on the way your "story" is developing. You can start with this one; it all depends on you, and how you think your partner would enjoy the kind of "story" you are about to tell!

The "A"
This basic "horny," or "hard" scenario starts with both palms facing away from you and the hands

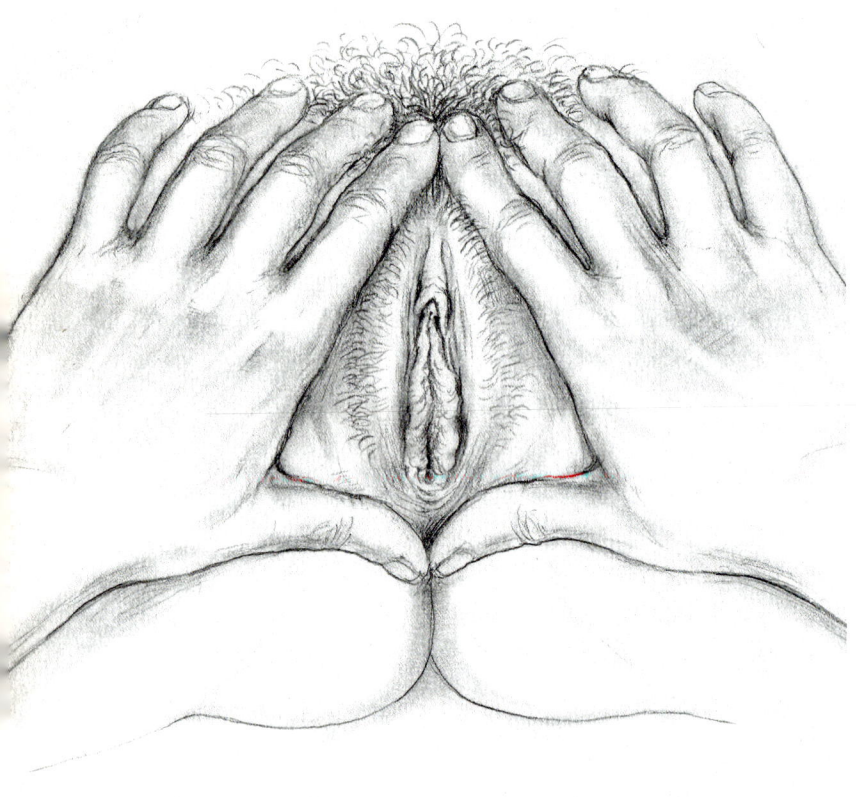

The 'A' Frame

brought together with only the forefingers and thumbs touching each other, the shape they make is a kind of "A". It also outlines the shape of the external female genitalia. This is easiest when her vulva is completely exposed, with her legs spread as far back or as wide as possible.

Placing this shape flat against the vulva with the palms on the inside of her thighs allows for a remarkable degree of control for your forefingers to squeeze or separate the top of the outer lips together. Later, you can come back to this, squeezing the top of the lips to expose the clitoral glans.

As you have to determine what works for you both, the next move may take a bit of practice: your thumbs can also (gently!) squeeze the lower part of both lips – or (gently!) separate them to expose the vaginal opening.

Utterly needless to add, your mouth

and tongue are at work at all times. Later, you can come back to this position, using your extended, stiff tongue to plunge in and out of the vagina. Remember to keep your teeth covered by your lips!

This particular use of your hands and tongue is made possible by her exposed position on her back. She will possibly need to help by holding her thighs wide apart, as your hands will be otherwise occupied.

But this can become tiring too, unless you're both fit or so consumed by paroxysms of lust that it doesn't seem to matter.

This position is, after all, one of the "dirtiest" or most "wanton" poses a female can make, especially when eye contact is maintained. We've left the Tantric, New Age or soft-lovey story here: this scene is pure down-and-dirty Boogie.

These basic hand positions can provide additional stimulation as well as allowing your mouth and tongue to move freely. Within both the "M" position as well as

CHECK OUT YOUR PERSONAL EQUIPMENT: LIPS

LIPS ARE THE 'PINCERS' of your oral equipment. Pull them back over your teeth and you'll have a very powerful pair of 'nippers' indeed. But they can equally supply that light touch needed at the start of operations. Push them out in a firm, rubbery pout or let them relax for a soft lip-to-lip landing. Open your mouth wide and envelop an area, then close down upon whatever might be there. Nibble, not with your teeth, but with your lips. Blow (upon the labia but NOT into the vagina – that's dangerous), suck, nip and nuzzle to your (and her) hearts' content.

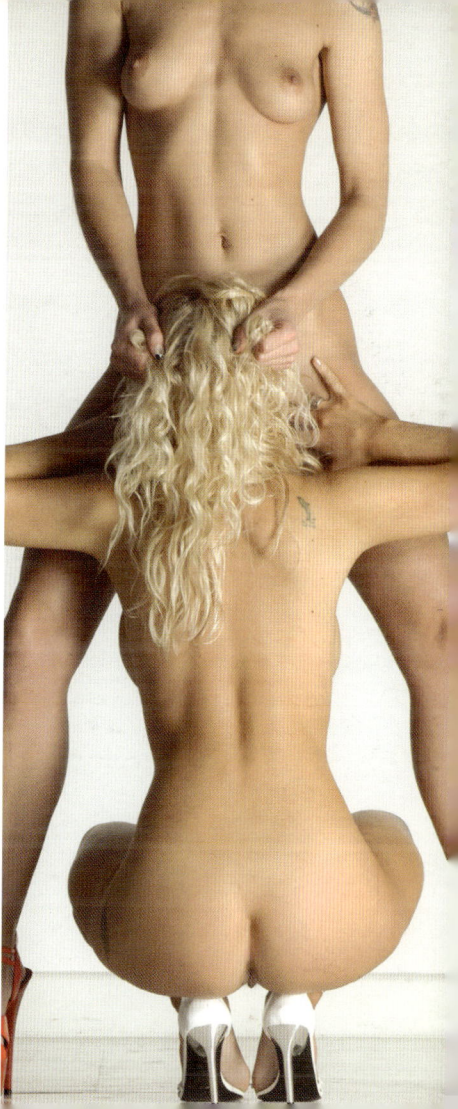

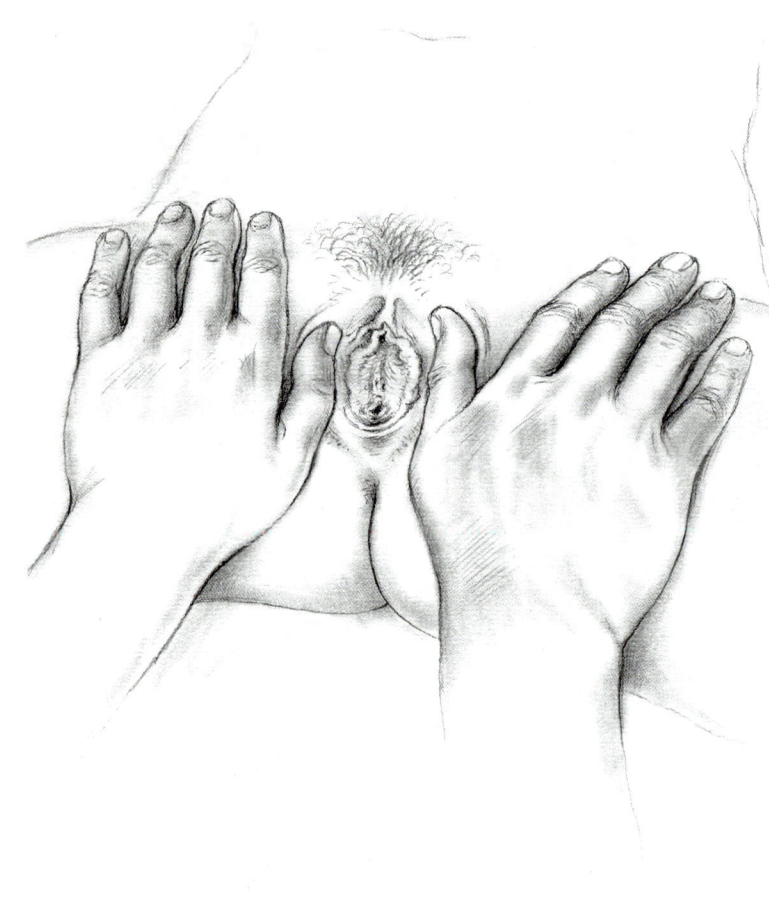

the "A" position, your hands have two interchangeable options:

The Spread
Gently spread first, the Labia Majora, or outer lips, with either your two forefingers (*opposite*) or thumbs (*this page*).

You don't want to touch the inner lips at this stage. The inner lips, as are the clitoris and the rest of her intimate erotic area, are extremely

THE FIVE SENSES: HEARING

THE SMALL, LIQUID SOUNDS that your tongue makes when sucking or licking between the folds of the pussy can be intensely erotic. But remember that cunnilingus is a partnership: it's essential to get feedback from the subject of your attentions; not a running commentary, perhaps, but it can be very rewarding if she lets you know you are pushing all the right buttons. Pure aural sex, really.

The Spread, with Thumbs
(this page)
The Spread, with Fingers
(opposite)

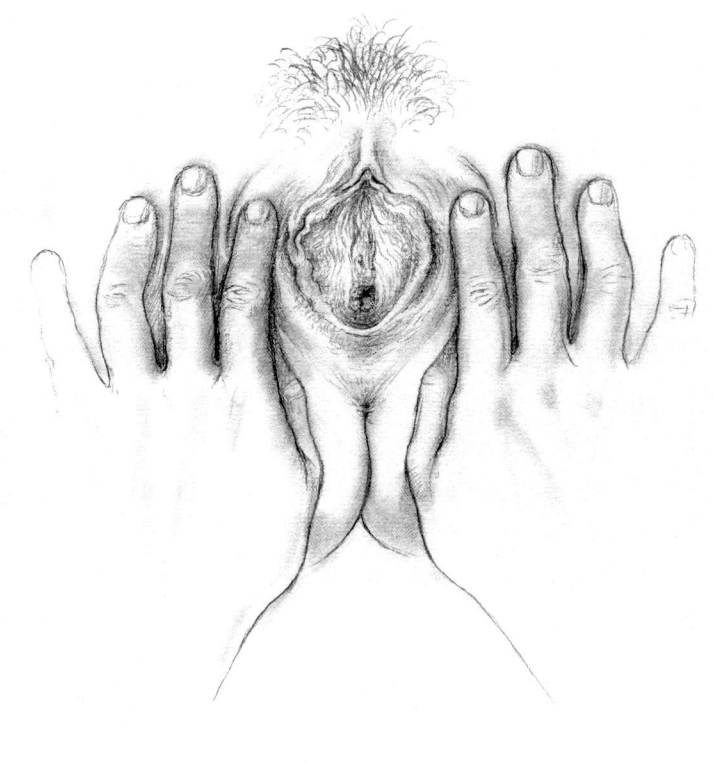

KRUG, PLEASE

"We had come to the end of an idyllic, slightly drunken picnic in the garden; it was one of those long summer afternoons that seem to go on for ever. We were both hot and there was still half a bottle of champagne in the cool bag. John got hold of the bottle and told me to take off my panties; at first I thought he was going to stick it up me and was about to tell him to desist in no uncertain terms, but he just trickled the cool fizzy liquid over my clit and labia as he sucked away. It was a really delicious feeling – and he was good enough to occasionally come up and share a mouthful of bubbly with me.."

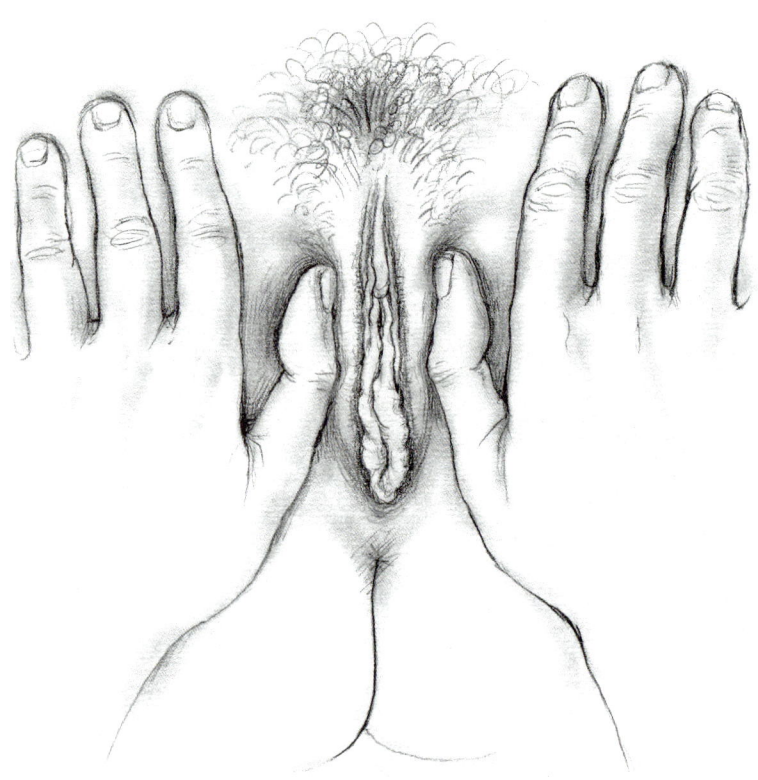

sensitive for many women at this point.

The Squeeze

"The Squeeze" is the reverse of "The Spread", and is a way of bringing the Labia Majora (the outer lips) together, either by gently stretching them at the top with your thumbs, or gently bringing them together with your forefingers.

"The Squeeze" allows the tip of your tongue, or the flat of your tongue, to play over the surface of the outer lips while your fingers maintain a gentle but firm tension in them. Not only can this heighten the sensation of pleasure, it has the advantage of letting her know more about the "story" you are "telling" her vulva with your mouth.

The clitoris is by now tumescent, and is sandwiched between both outer lips – whatever its size. Be aware that with some women the clitoris can be actually peeking slightly above the outer labial fold.

The Squeeze, with Thumbs (this page)
The Squeeze, with Fingers (opposite)

At this stage you still want to play "house odds" by avoiding it with the rough part of your tongue. It may still be too sensitive for direct contact.

The pressure of your mouth and tongue on the taut labia will be both

CHECK OUT YOUR PERSONAL EQUIPMENT: MOUTH AND TEETH

"TEETH? ARE YOU CRAZY?" you might ask. Well, teeth can intensify the 'nibble' effect that the lips provide and you can even press your bared teeth gently against various parts of the vulva to provide a very different sensation. Then the whole mouth itself can be used - as a musical instrument: humming produces pleasantly strong vibrations (hence 'hum job'). And opening wide and drawing in the whole of your loved one's soft parts can be a beautiful way of expressing love and tenderness towards her.

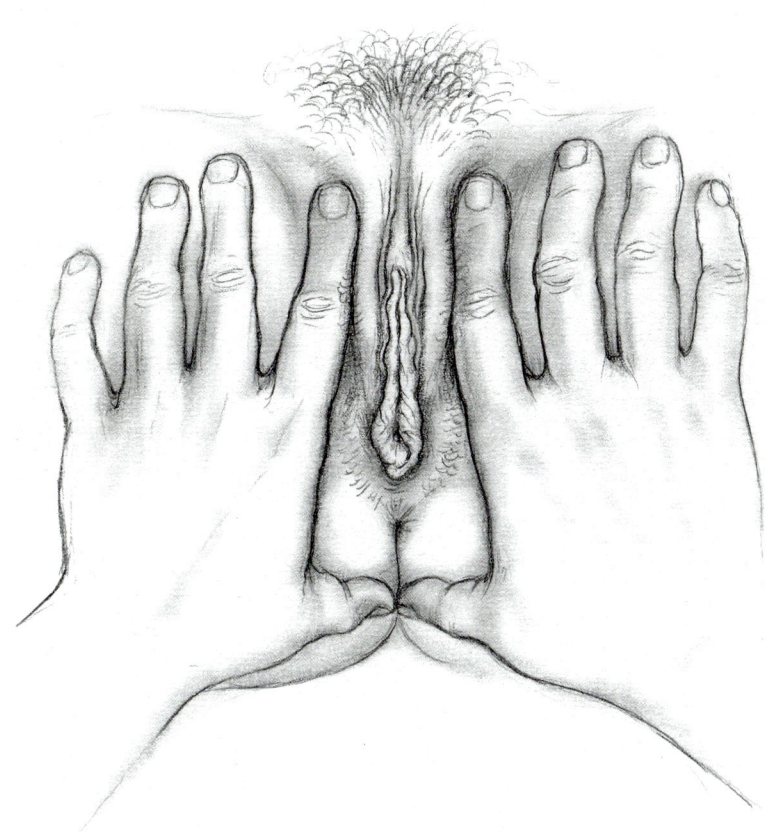

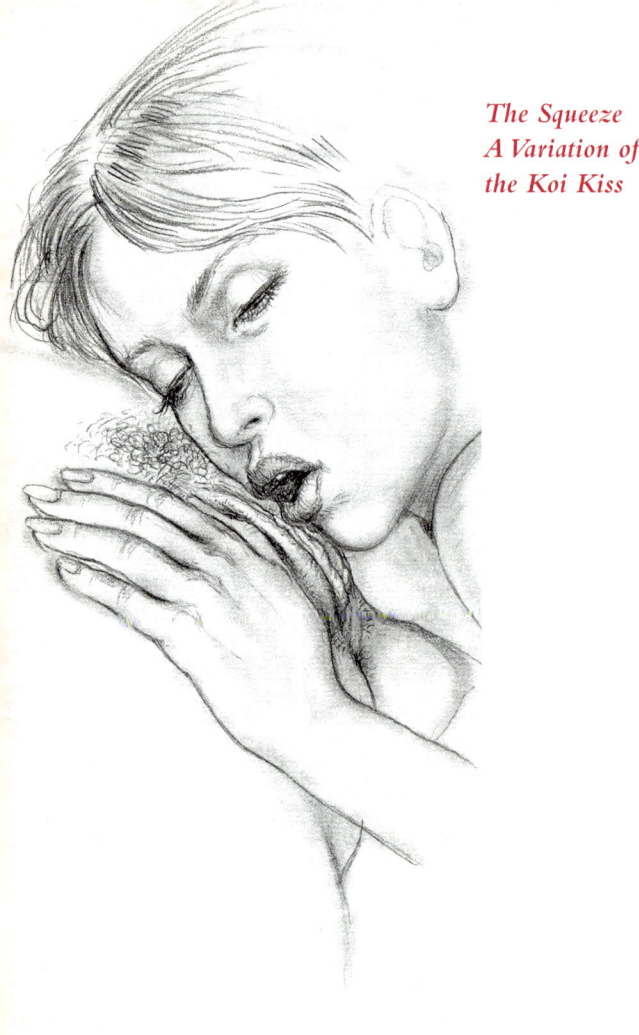

The Squeeze
A Variation of the Koi Kiss

physically and mentally stimulating, especially with the added variation of turning your head slightly to the side and opening and closing your lips on them in a variation of the Koi Kiss (see Chapter 4).

Many women appreciate the additional stimulation of a finger or fingers inserted into the vagina and/or anus (anal stimulation appealing to some, but by no means all), while giving head at the same time. If this is the first cunnilingual experience in your relationship, even the most experienced women appreciate this additional stimulation introduced tentatively.

Why tentatively? For two reasons: First, it cannot be repeated too often that the vast range of responses available to women can change from day to day, and even from minute to minute. Areas can become sensitive. Needs can flip from "Do it hard!" to "Gently! Gently!" without warning. The best lovers are aware of this at all

THE FIVE SENSES: SMELL

MOST ARDENT CUNNILINGUISTS rave about the intoxicating, musky smell that women exude when they are wet and sexually excited, signalling a sexual urgency that simply cannot be ignored. Other enthusiasts wax lyrical about a whole range of natural olfactory delights such as exotic, spicy sandalwood, new-mown hay or fresh, clean sea breeze. But then there's the fishy thing, too, and that's when some react with, "I'm worried I don't smell very nice." Solution? Just rinse with a little warm water before sex and the intensity of odour should reduce to a very acceptable level. But if your pussy persists in smelling pretty awful then again, it could be time for a visit to your gynie. Some swear that cranberry juice (you drink it by the way, don't try douching) is the answer to the sweetest smelling pussy. No harm in trying.

times, and the best lovers help their best lovers by keeping them informed.

And, moreover, the vast range of responses available to the female don't all turn on, like Christmas lights, at the flick of a switch. Some zones warm up here; some thoughts get excited there; and never forget that in most cases, the last to turn on is the clitoris itself.

You don't have to have a big discussion about it: your tentative (but not timid) movements and the responses of your partner will tell you which way you both want to go.

It's not what you can do; it's how you do it and with whom you do it with, which marks the superior lover from the show-off, and (however energetic) the well-meaning but boring.

Back to the hands. The simultaneous insertion of a finger

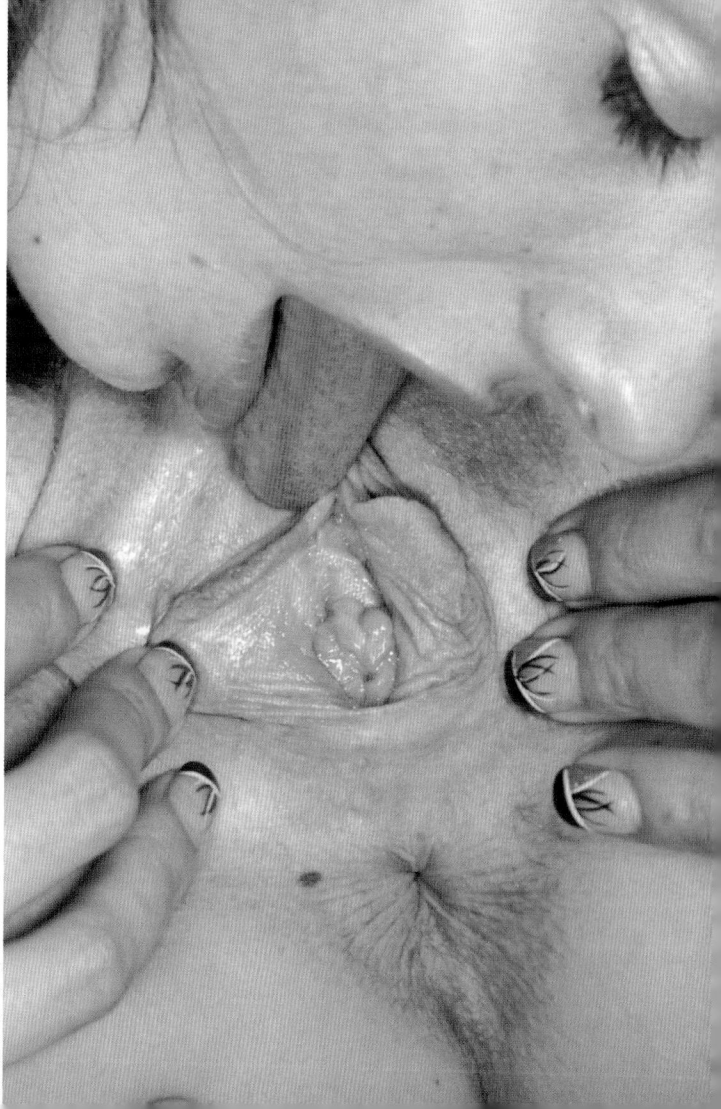

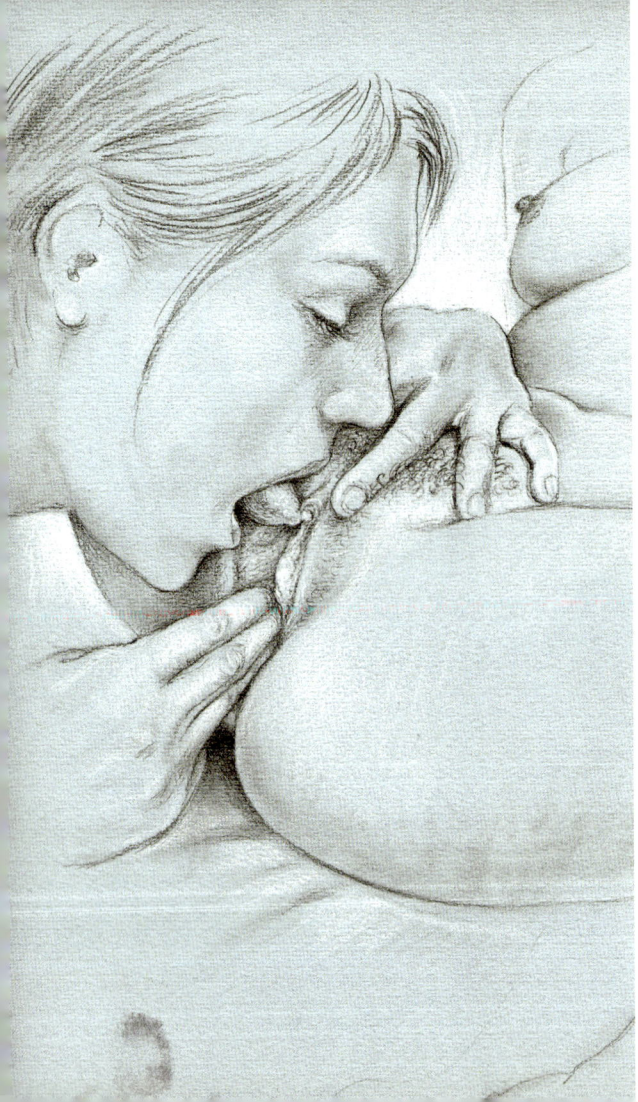

into the vagina during cunnilingus can appear to be a bit awkward, in that the natural direction of the finger in this position will be curving downward, thus making the "beckoning" stimulation of the G-spot difficult.

But stimulation of the G-spot certainly need not always be a consequence of finger-fucking. Some women respond to the G-spot thing, and some don't. But with a little perseverance and proper stimulation most can, and will.

At any rate, the fingers can of course be inserted curving upwards in order to stimulate the periurethral sponge and the G-spot. Just be sure that any change in positions is initially gentle.

Before we look at G-spot technique, let's look at some of the "stories" the fingers can "tell".

How does she masturbate? If you've

EMOTIONS AND PSYCHOLOGY

"THERE'S NO DIFFERENCE between a blow job and going down", you might argue, but there is. A woman is stripping herself naked both literally and emotionally when she opens herself up to you for cunnilingus. Of course some are confident enough to relax and enjoy it all, perhaps even indulging in their favourite fantasies that might not involve you at all. Others get quite a buzz out of the power trip it can provide, relishing the fact that they are in the position of authority, directing you with their hands on your head or simply telling you what to do. But for some women the feeling of vulnerability and exposure can be extreme – especially if it's the first time – and male partners should advance with tenderness and sensitivity. Tongue Talking will always help to bridge the gap.

Using Fingers as a Cone
(opposite page)

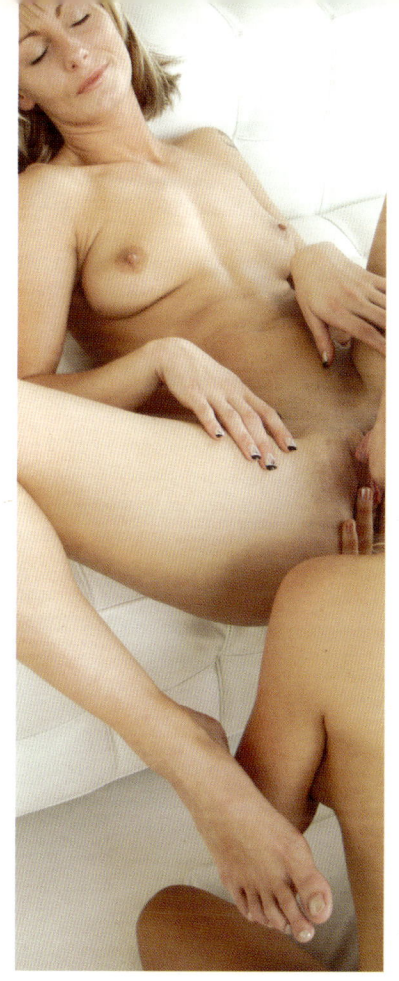
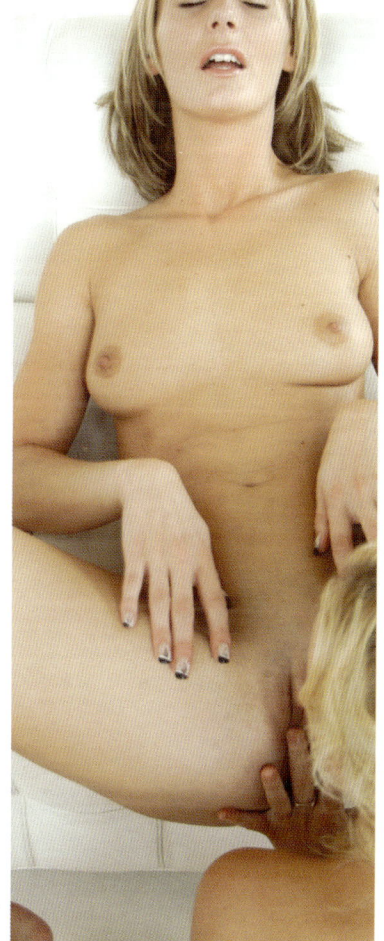

GREAT KISSERS

"Men who kiss me really well, passionately, creatively, greedily, as if they can't quite get enough of me are usually brilliant at going down on me, too. It's a little test I use and I don't think I've been proved wrong yet. Kissing someone on the lips is a great indicator of what's to come, so I never skip that stage."

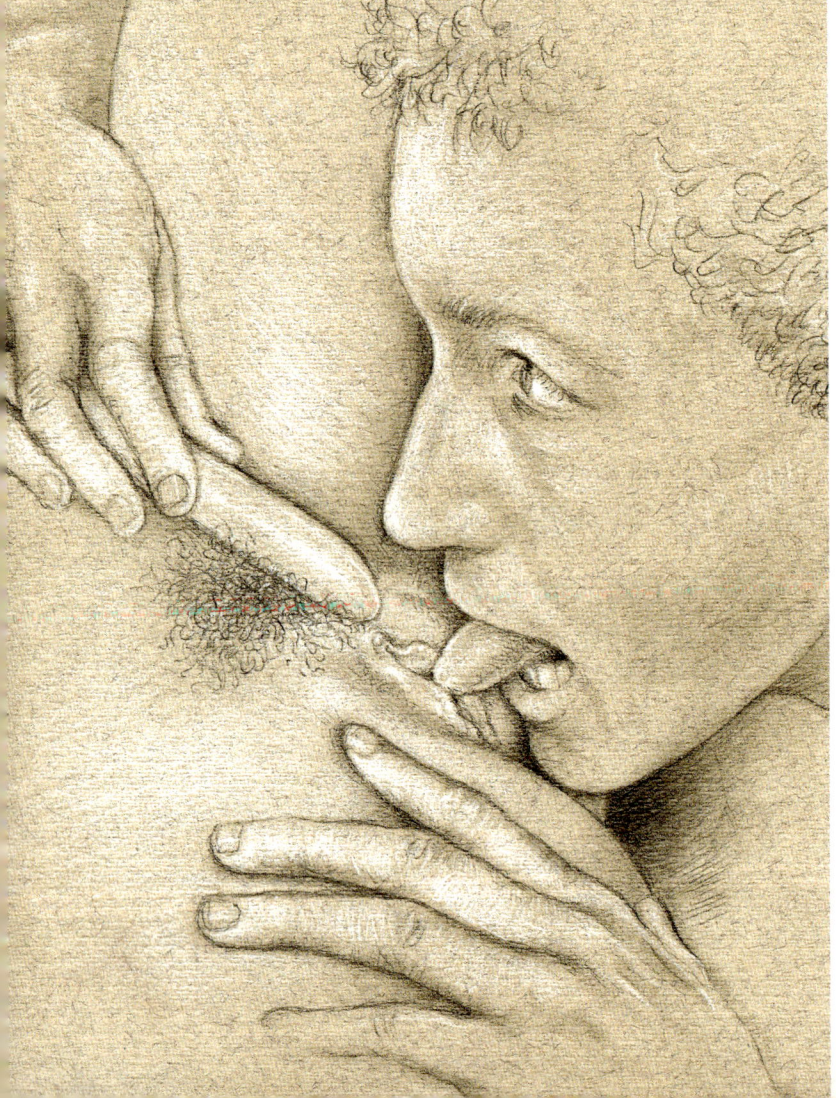

had a chance to observe, do it the way she does it. You will notice that 99% of the time the clitoral glans is never directly stimulated. Usually a finger down the side of it brings the best response.

And how you do it certainly counts as "storytelling". If she likes talk or fantasies (the subject of another book), a little narration as you wank her can go a long way.

One or more fingers gently probe the inside of the vagina, and pull out very slowly, as if asking the silent, teasing question: Do you want more? You don't need to wait for an answer; if you've got your timing right, her vulva is already nodding up and down in agreement.

Two fingers can be pushed in stiff and held there while she moves around on them, after which they can spread apart on either side of the urethral sponge with a gentle "let your fingers do the walking" motion.

The Pocket Rocket

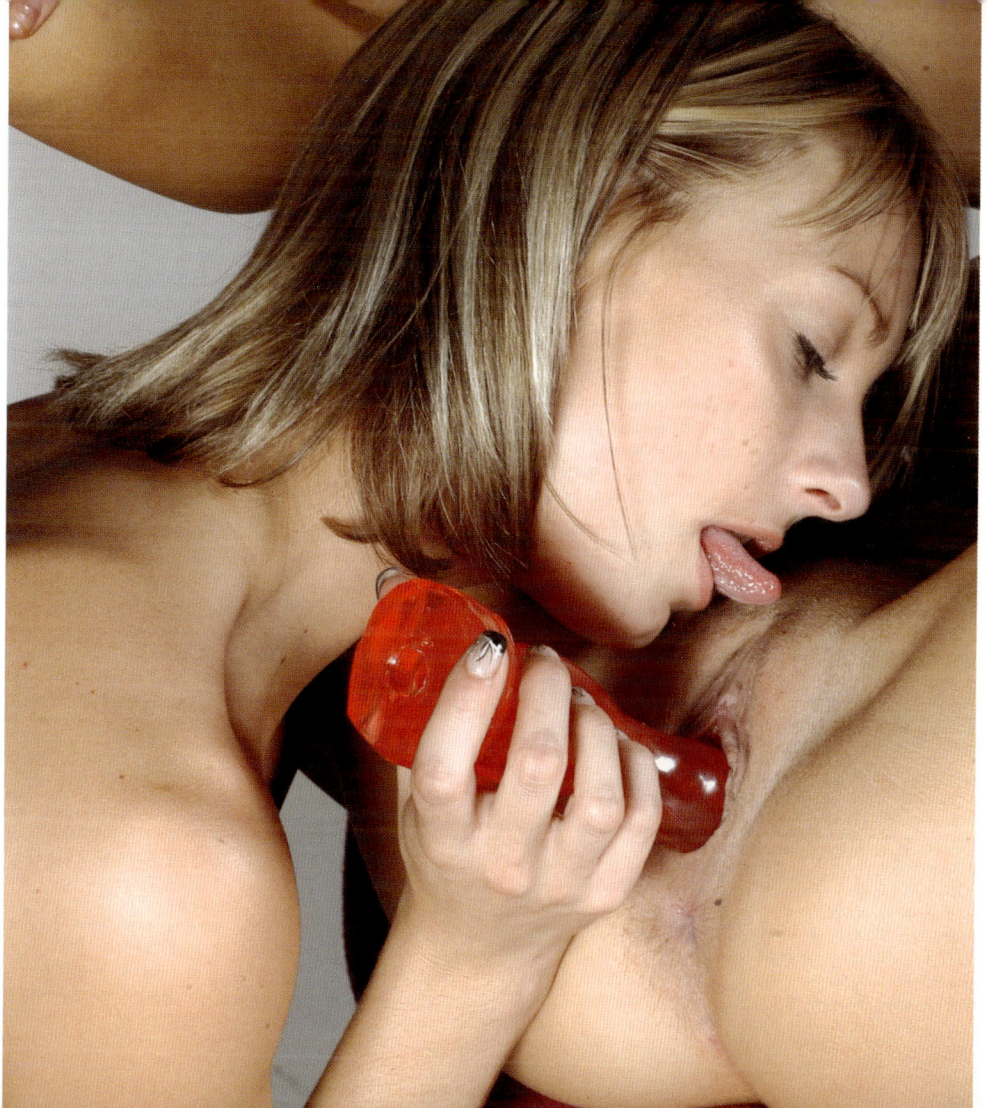

Three fingers can be shaped into a cone like a butt-plug, letting your partner move around on them, letting you know if this is just right, or too much.

With a latex glove, two fingers can go up to the knuckle and the back of the fingers can rub either side of the periurethral sponge. Latex gloves can be included as one of many "perverse" touches you can employ should you wish to take your "story" into fantasy (or fanny-teasy, as one of our "perverse" friends puts it).

As well as adding that touch of Doctor-and-Patient "perversity", latex gloves can provide protection against scratching and any possibilities of infection, or, just as important, anxieties about both.

Coordination of fingers and mouth may seem a bit like rubbing your stomach and patting your head, but you can take comfort that, with this particular art, practice is never a chore.

Other Devices

Cunnilingus, as discussed briefly here, is primarily about the lips and tongue, but we cannot ignore hands or positions. There remains the idea of devices, such as the use of a current favourite sex-toy, the "Pearl Rabbit", which incorporates revolving beads, a clitoral stimulator and dildo in one battery-operated vibrator.

Vibrating dildos come in a variety of sizes and widths. They can be single or double, that is, where both the vagina and the rectum are penetrated. Use of these should be agreed on in advance – whether hours before or on the spot is up to you; the only point is not to surprise your partner with something unfamiliar and perhaps not liked. But a discussion of vibrators, restraints, etc. takes the action beyond the scope of this book.

However two "extras" will get a

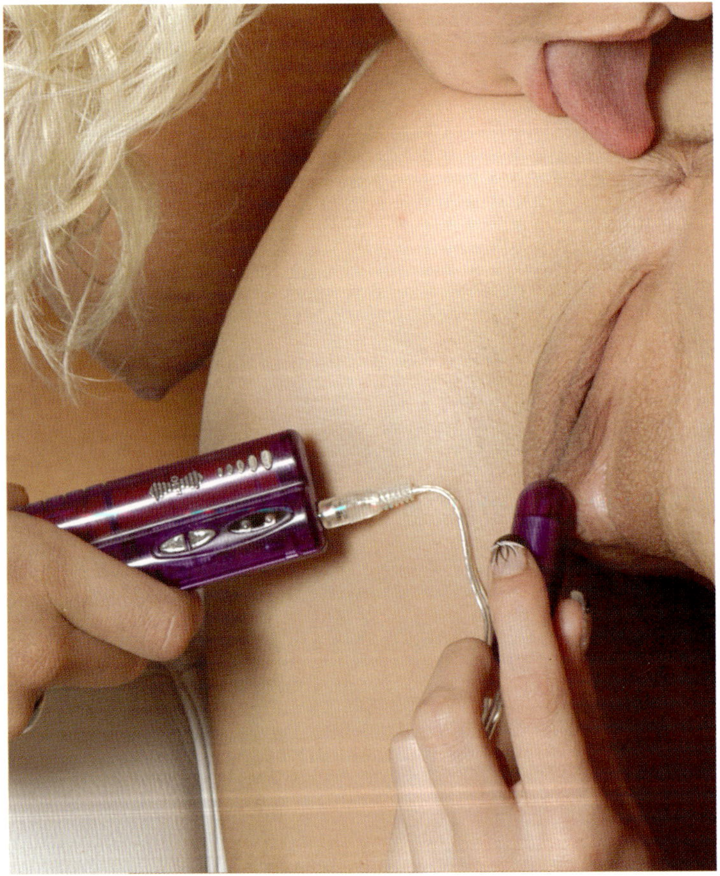

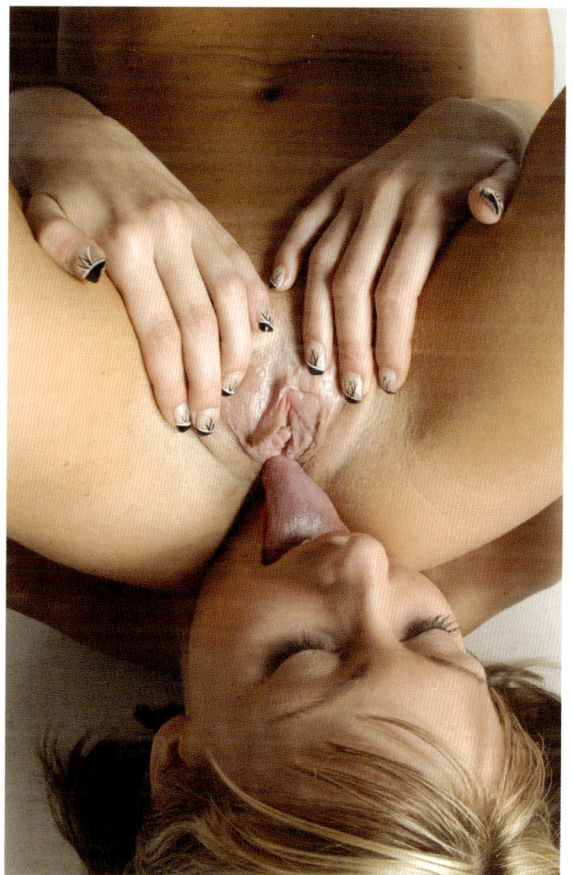

brief mention:

Cling-film is not only a great safety barrier; it can be a real turn on. If you haven't tried it, don't knock it – yet. Cling-film is on the edge of fantasy; it has the same function as fur-lined hand-cuffs: it plays with the idea of restraint.

The "pocket rocket" vibrator, applied just above the clitoral glans is a great way to provide additional stimulation at the same time as the mouth and tongue. These little buzzers are more powerful than they look, so it might be a good idea to introduce it over and around the pubic bone first.

All these suggestions can be applied (with some modification) to any sexual position, some of which will be discussed in the following chapter.

BRINGING TOYS TO THE PARTY

WHETHER IT'S A VIBRATOR, your electric toothbrush, a butt plug or strong peppermint or ice cubes in the mouth, you can very easily liven up an already great act with these accoutrements. Tongue Joy and The Bedside Bullet (see pages 62, 81) are just two of the increasingly sophisticated toys you can now buy - visit the EPS website (www.eroticprints.org) for more details.

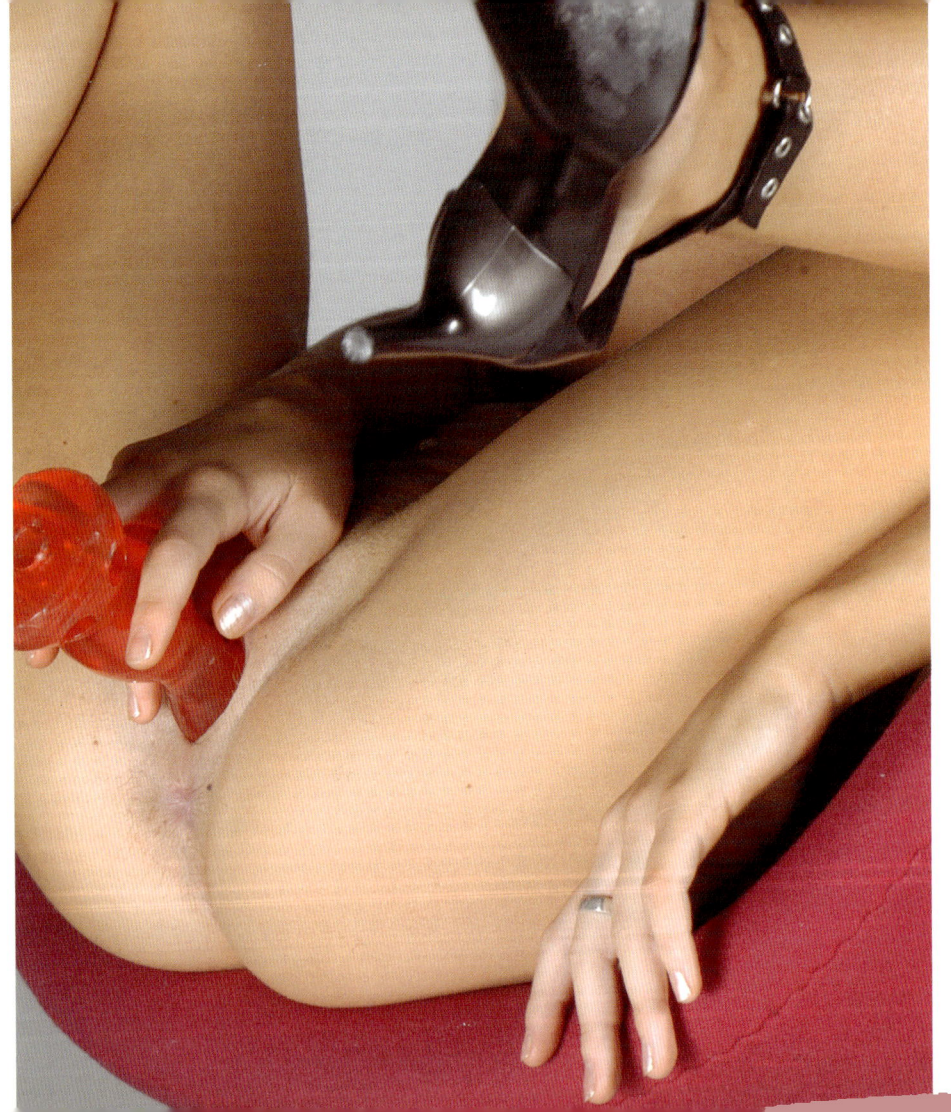

VI BODY POSITIONS

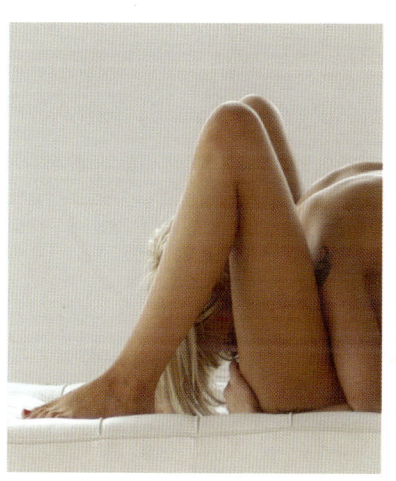 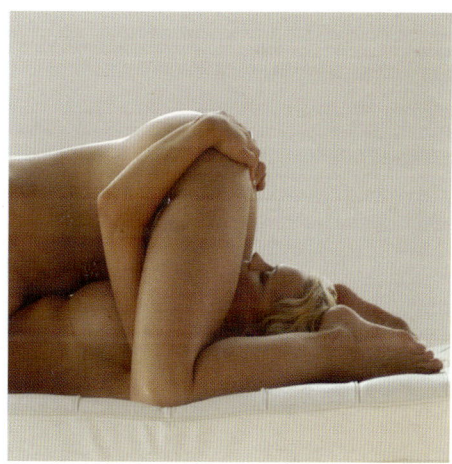

There are as many positions in which to enjoy cunnilingus as any other sexual activity; they all have the power to excite and amplify an already charged scenario. We've already looked at the most common position, and now we'll discuss three others. They are:

1. Le Sixty-Nine
The possibilities for stimulation and "story" obviously change when matters turn upside-down. Her buttocks are above and on

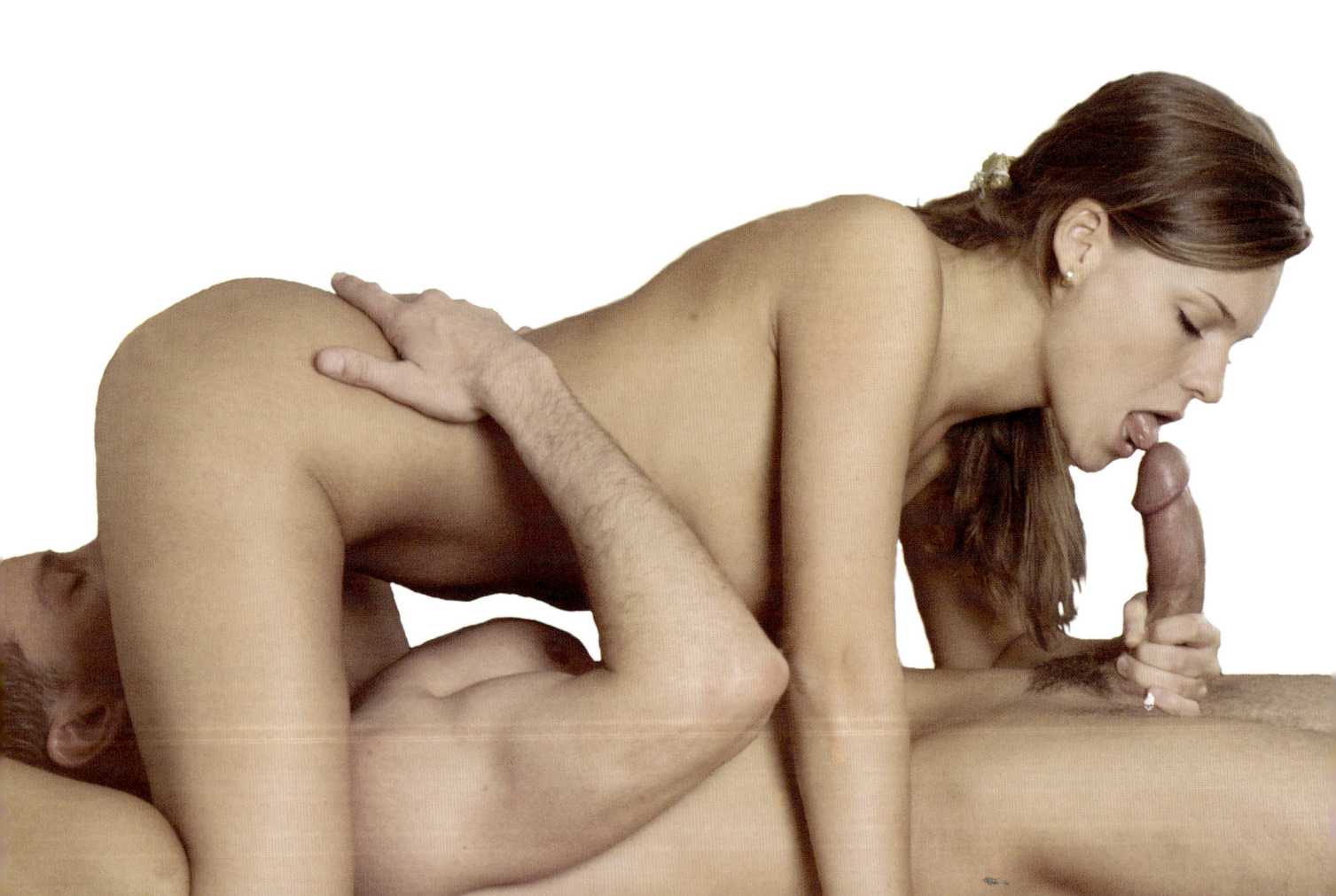

Buttock Play

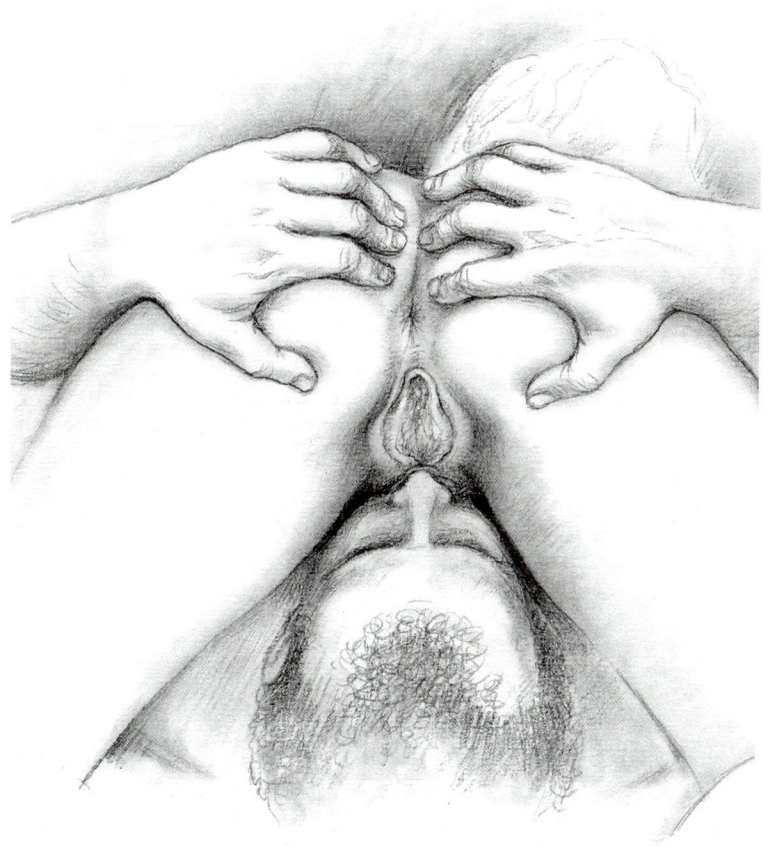

top of you, and this necessitates a considerable physical change in tongue technique.

Your teeth are now a greater hazard than in the "missionary" position, on the edge of a bed or chair or standing facing you. And your chin now comes into play as never before, as her pubic bone is next to, it if not on top of, it.

But your partner has more control here over how closely, how fast and how much she receives oral sex. I say "receive," but muffled shouts of "Fuck my face!" can call this verb into question more often than not…

So, making sure your teeth don't accidentally scrape the underside of her clitoral glans and your chin doesn't bang too hard against her pubic bone, and (for men) your face is (for those who don't like beards) shaved as clean and smooth as it can be, you are left with your mouth and tongue (whose

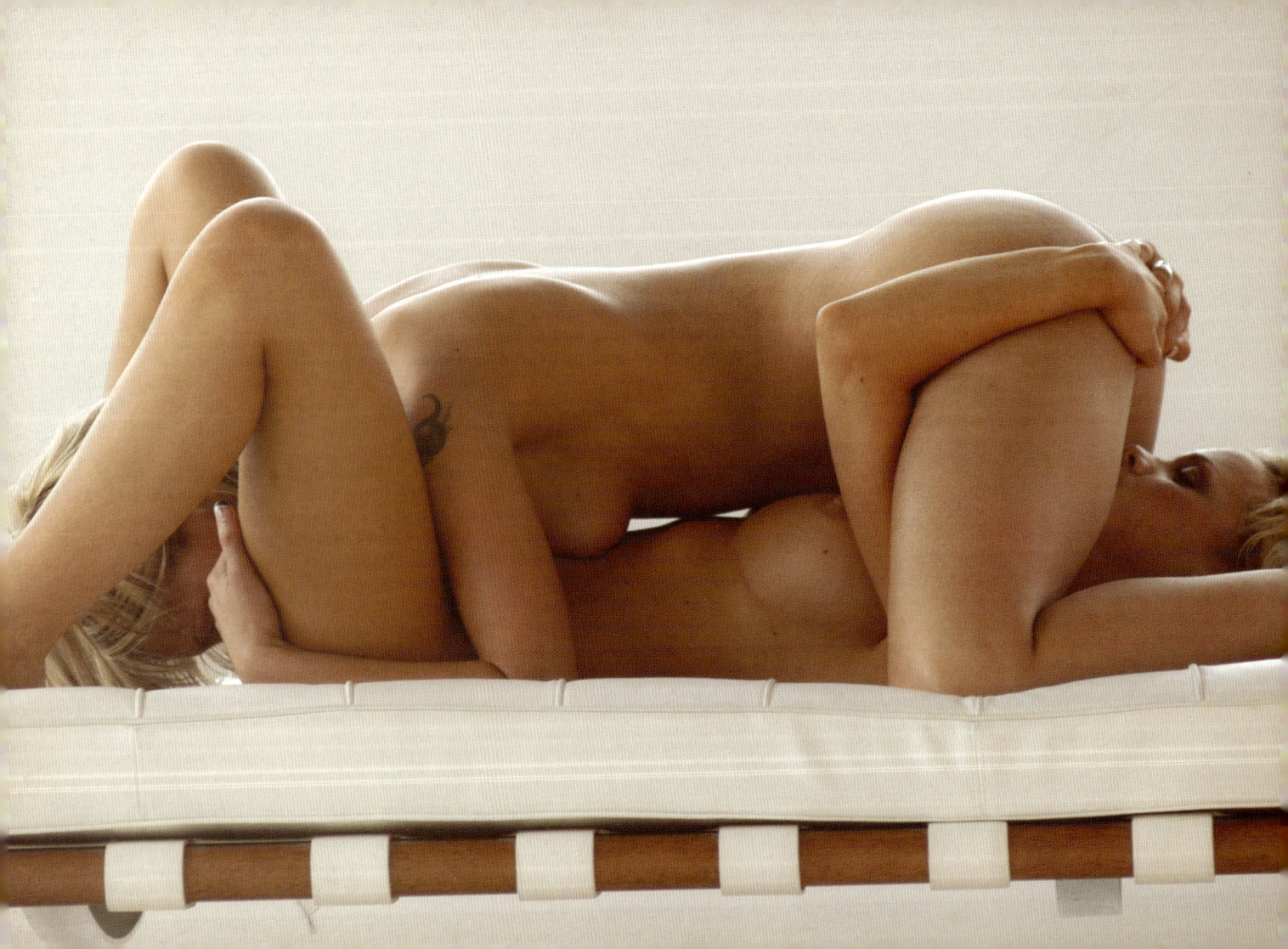

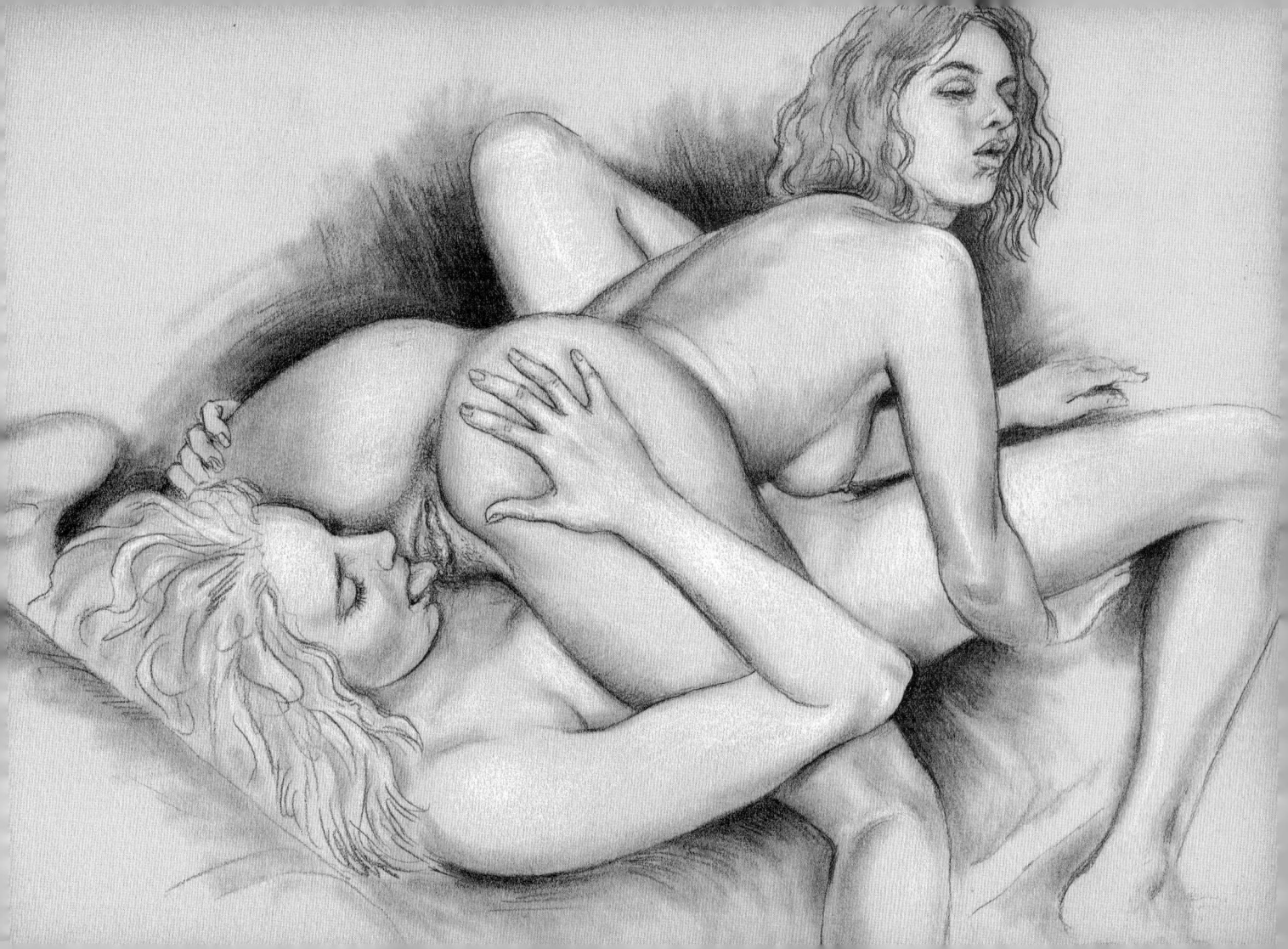

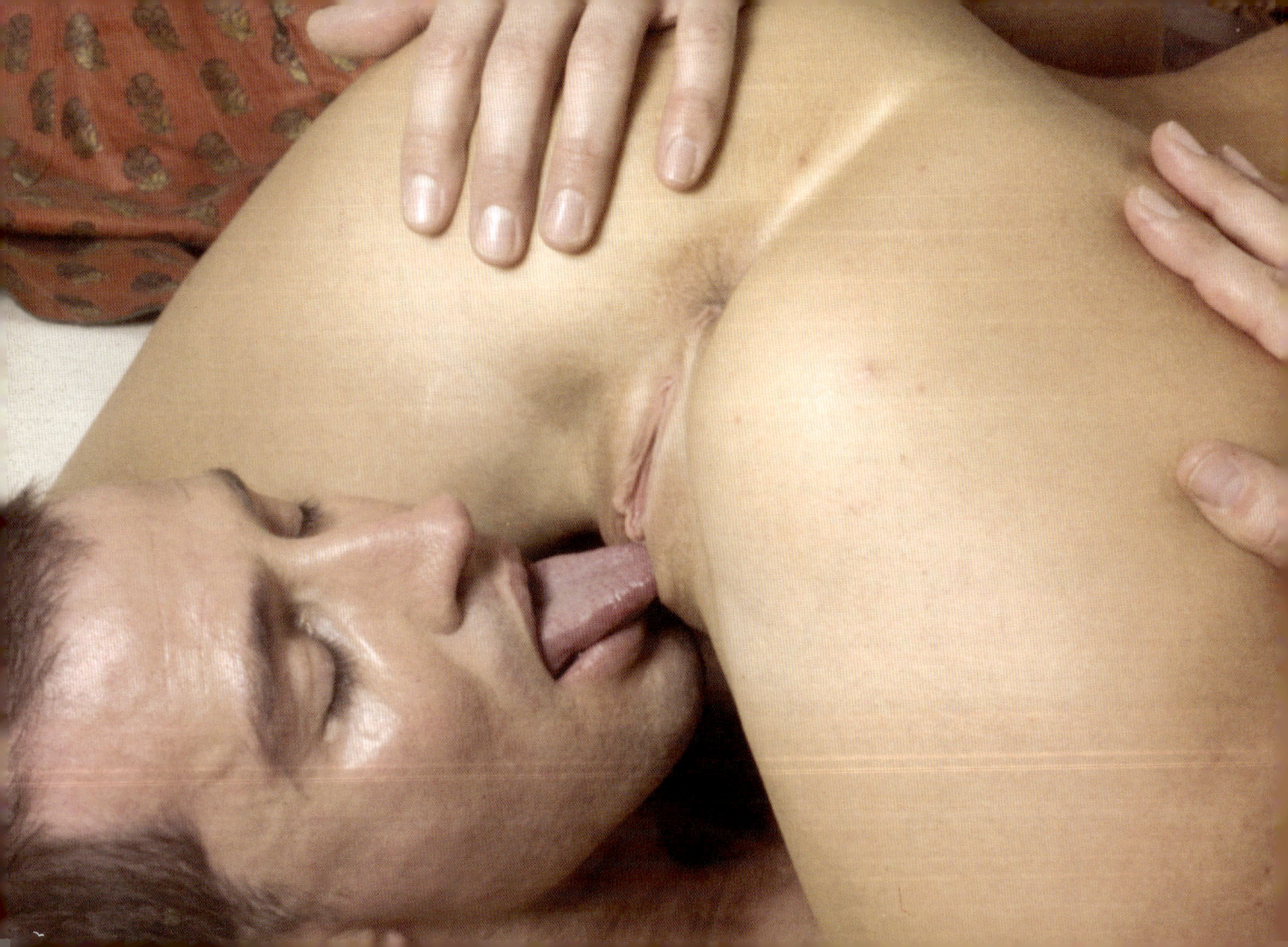

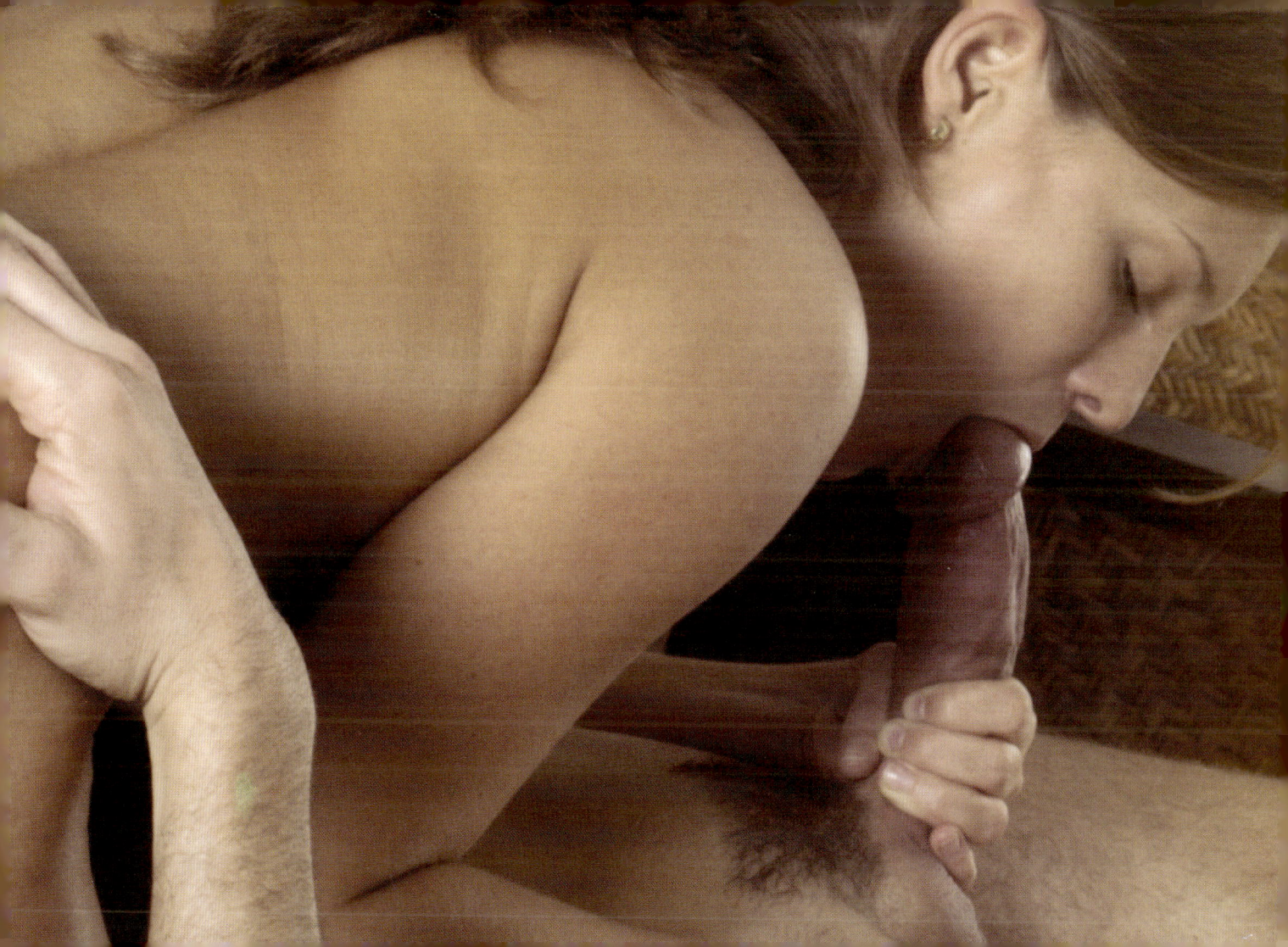

frenulum will now be sorely tested), and your hands.

Here is where buttock-play comes into its own. If you like your partner's buttocks (and why shouldn't you?), the way you stroke, caress, knead or squeeze them will let her know it, and if you ever wanted proof of your sexual originality or creativity, however attenuated or limited you thought it to be, here is where you will find it in yourself. Any outside clues or suggestions here will only spoil your sense of discovery.

Here, too, the line between emotional-sensual and down-and-dirty-sensual is clearer than in other positions. There are no rules which say you have to stick with one scenario or the other; all you have to remember is not to work the changes mechanically, i.e. "by numbers."

Let's be frank about it: in this position your partner is willingly exposing, even exhibiting, her

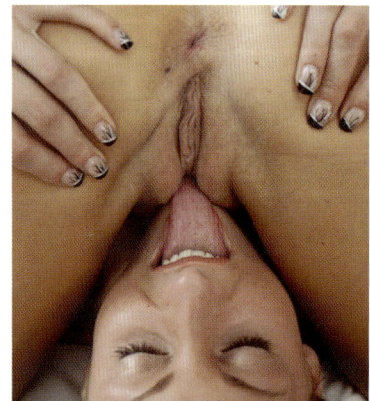
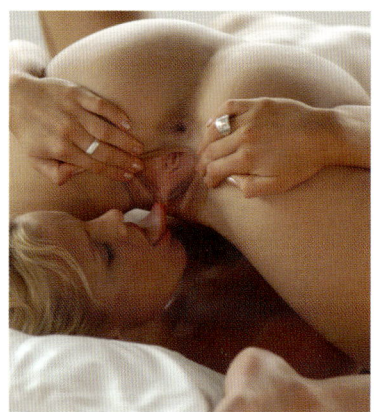
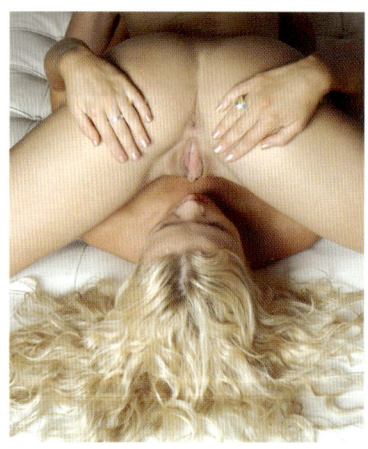
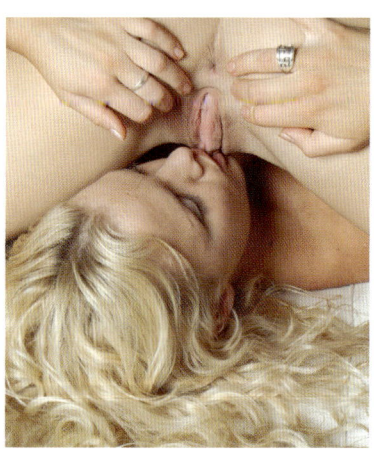

Soixante Neuf, Girl-Boy *(this page)*
Soixante Neuf, Girl-Girl *(page 69)*

intimate parts to you without the mental safety net of being able to look down and check your response, and without being able to communicate verbally or guide your head with her hands. Her daringly vulnerable position implies "the ball is in your court", and a good opening response is to make some vulnerable moves yourself.

One example is to pull her closer, as if acknowledging the awkwardness of the intimacy, and your desire to overcome it. Your neck muscles will need to support the movements of your head as, with your hands now spreading her vulva open, your tongue, stretched to its limit, thrusts deeply in and out of her vagina. A helpful pillow beneath your head is not cheating.

But, down-and-dirty or no, with "Sixty-Nine" many women feel ambivalent about being able to "let go completely" if they're also involved in giving pleasure as well.

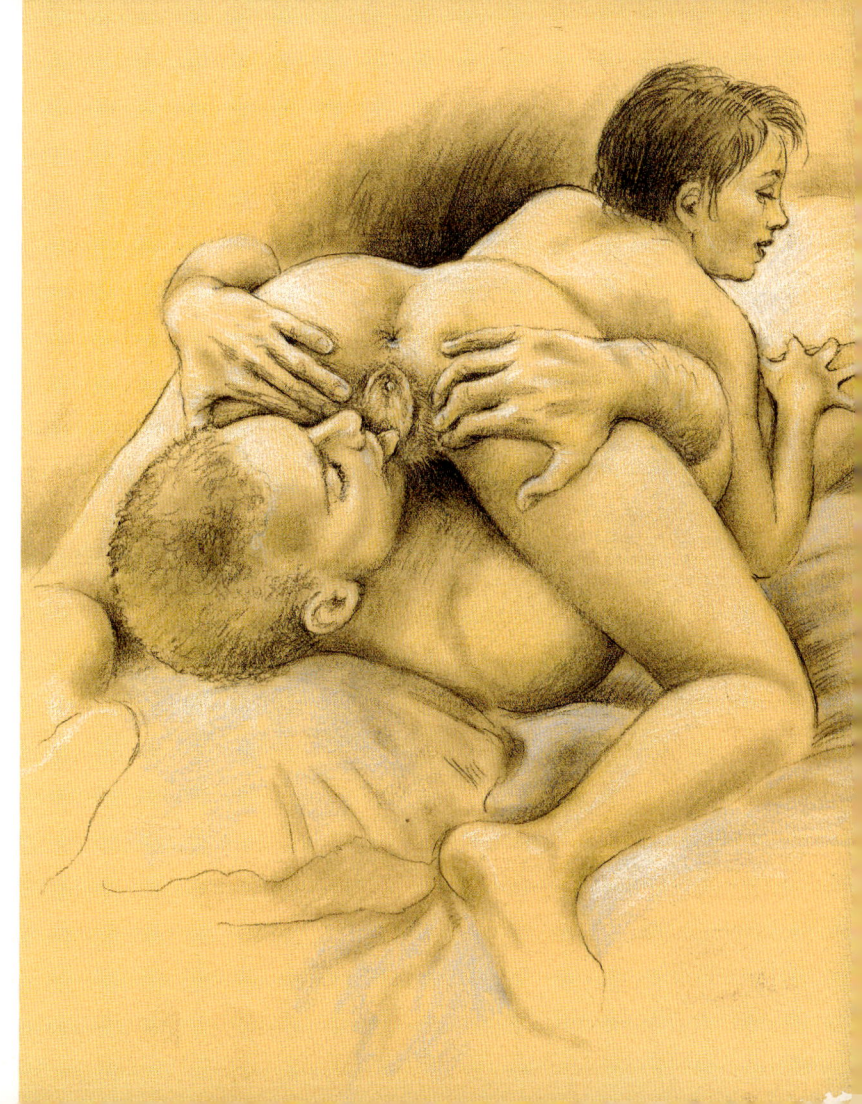

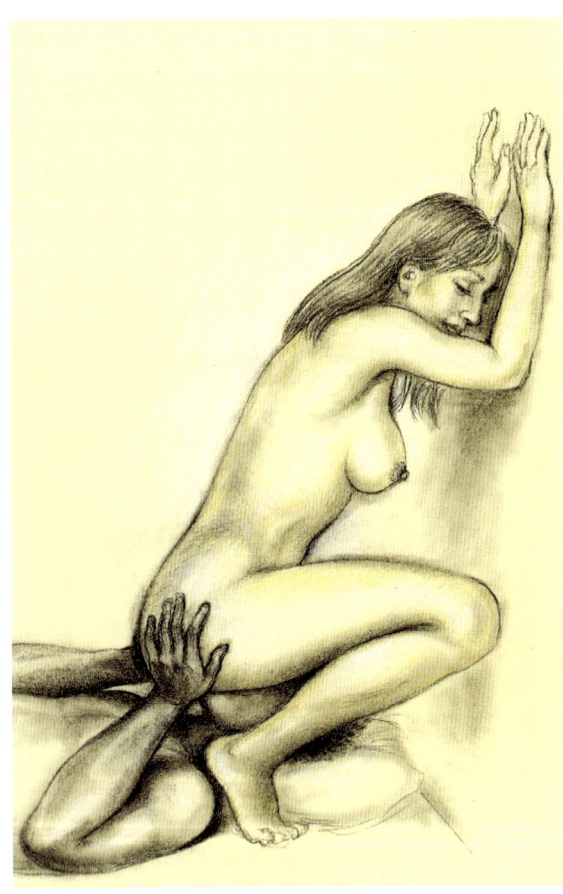

If things get too rough (teeth), a cry of "Gently!" accompanied by a reassuring squeeze will not halt proceedings. This goes for both parties.

Many women respond to the "head-trip" of sixty-nine, and are able to experience very different (but no less intense) kinds of orgasms.

2. Face-Sitting
(1) This is where the woman straddles the face of the cunnilinguist. She can now look down, brace her hands against a wall or on either side of her partner's head; in other words, take charge of the oral sex, or "use" the face of her partner to tell her own "story." She can add to the situation with her own hands or with a vibrator. And she can warn her partner if she is about to ejaculate when she comes.

(2) She can also turn and face the other way, bracing her hands

Face Sitting
with vibrator
(opposite)
Face Sitting
(this page)

DOMINATRICE

"There's definitely a submissive side to me and I find it extraordinarily sexy to lie there while my partner, who has a lovely large, hairy pussy with very protruding inner lips, slowly descends upon my face. I often wait until her labia are touching my lips. It's an incredible feeling and sometimes I heighten it by getting her to put some restraints on my wrists so that I'm more or less helpless as she does this. Then she just rocks her pelvis on my mouth until she comes and I get almost drowned in her juices – the bit I love best of all."

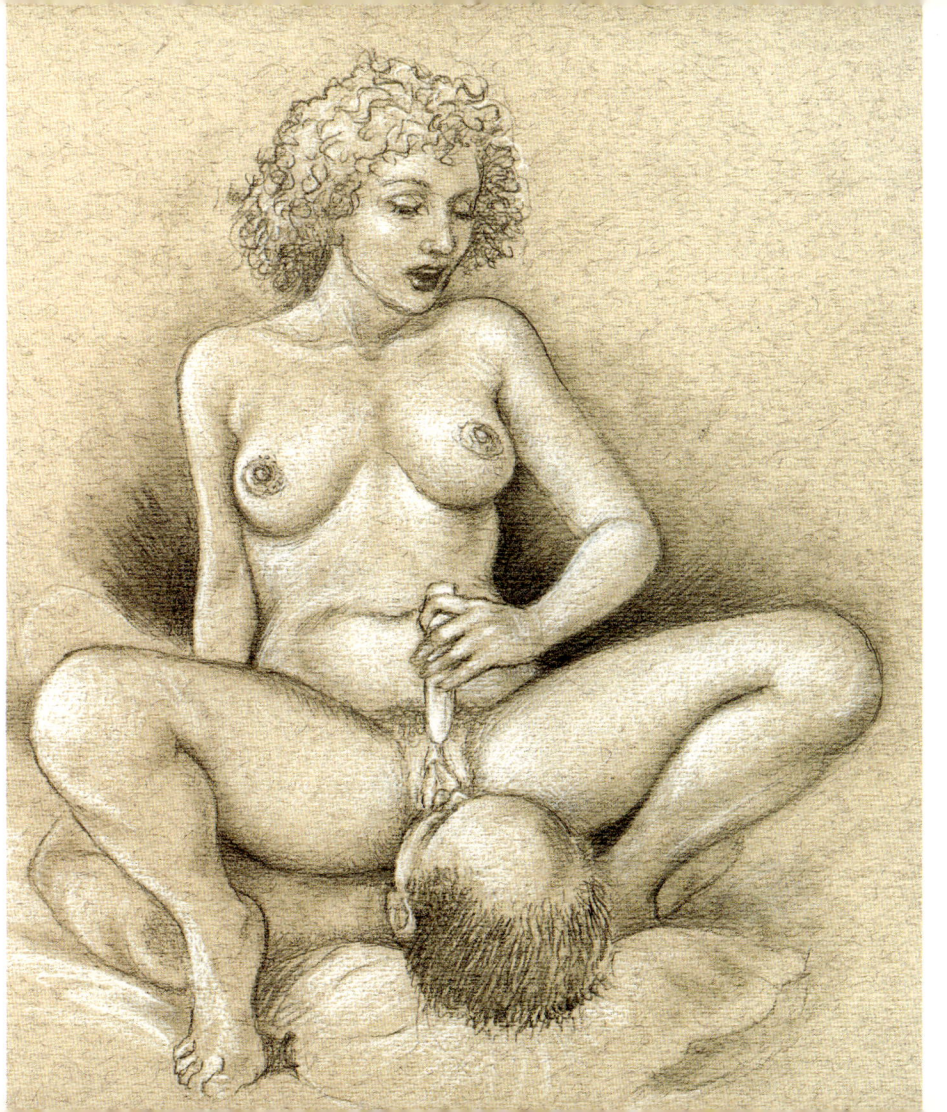

WATCH YOUR LANGUAGE

THEY MAY ONLY BE WORDS but they have a huge potency that is not always recognised. The C-word, especially. "Your cunt is really yummy!" or "Suck my cunt harder, you lazy, no-good fucker!" might be pure audial aphrodisia to some, but could horrify others. Earthy talk and going down are usually good bed partners, but it's as well to go easy, even though the context of sex and intimacy would seem a good place to use bad language of the sexual kind. Establish what words you like in advance – then let it rip. Otherwise it could be the premature end of a beautiful relationship.

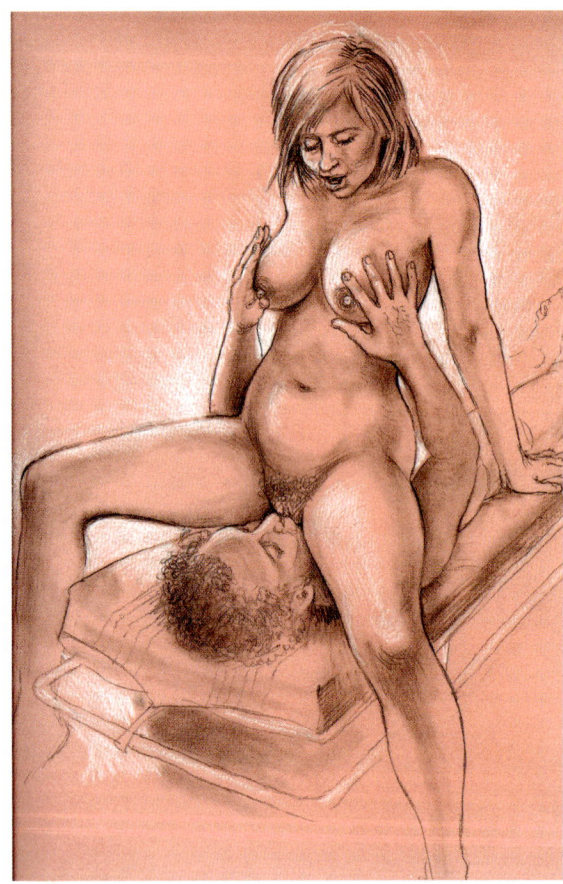

Face Sitting, Crouching Over (opposite)
Face Sitting, Leaning Back (this page)

CUPBOARD LOVE

"I'm not sure why, but I find the kitchen a really erotic place to make love; it's the heart of our house and perhaps it brings out the sensuous, Nigella-type in me, but I've often bent over our big, rustic pine table with my jeans down or laid back on it with my skirt up while my partner feasts on me from behind or in front; I love cooking and lots of different tastes and textures, so I always get him to put a finger in my mouth after he's been playing with my pussy. I often joke that if he makes me come I'll cook him one of his favourites..."

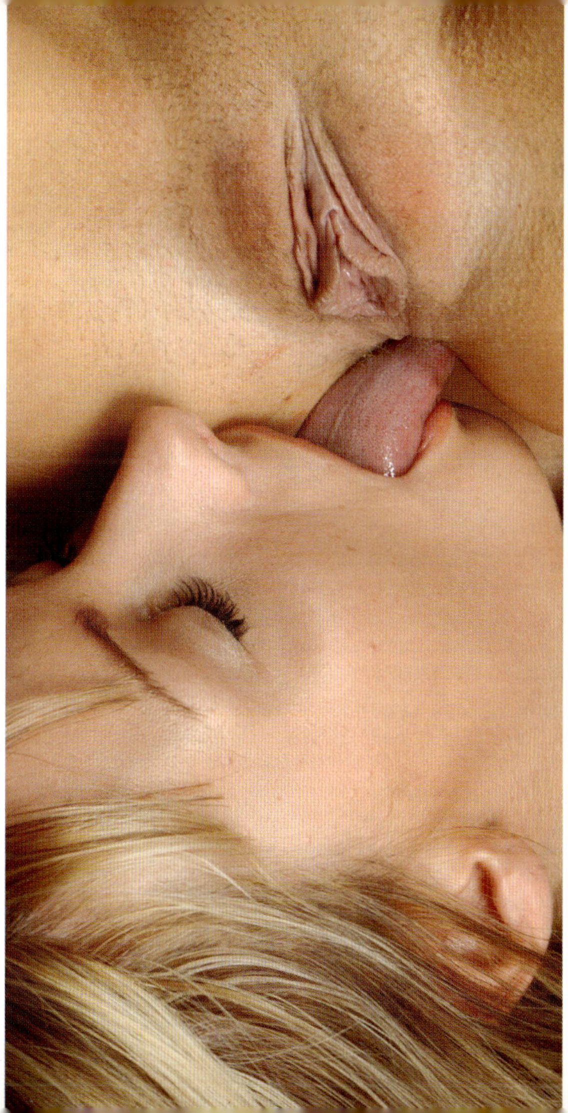

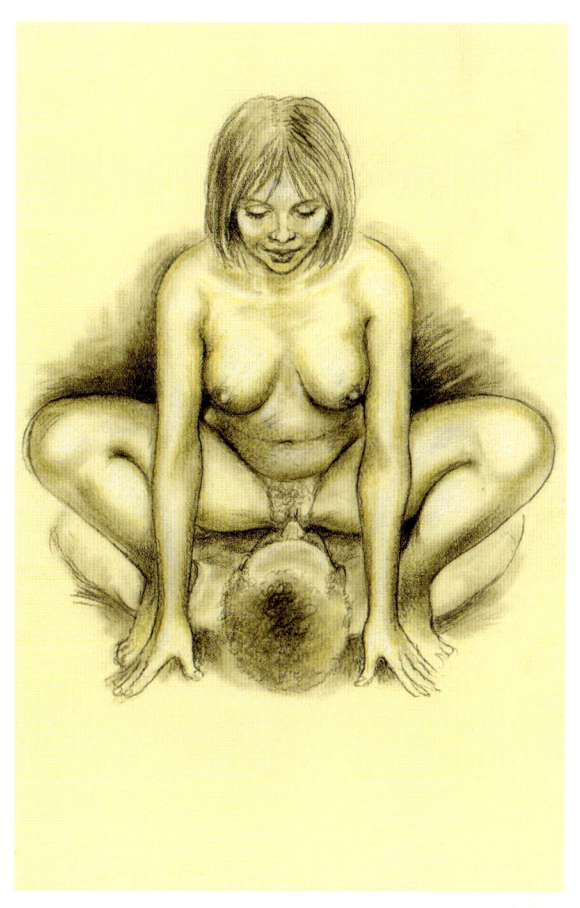

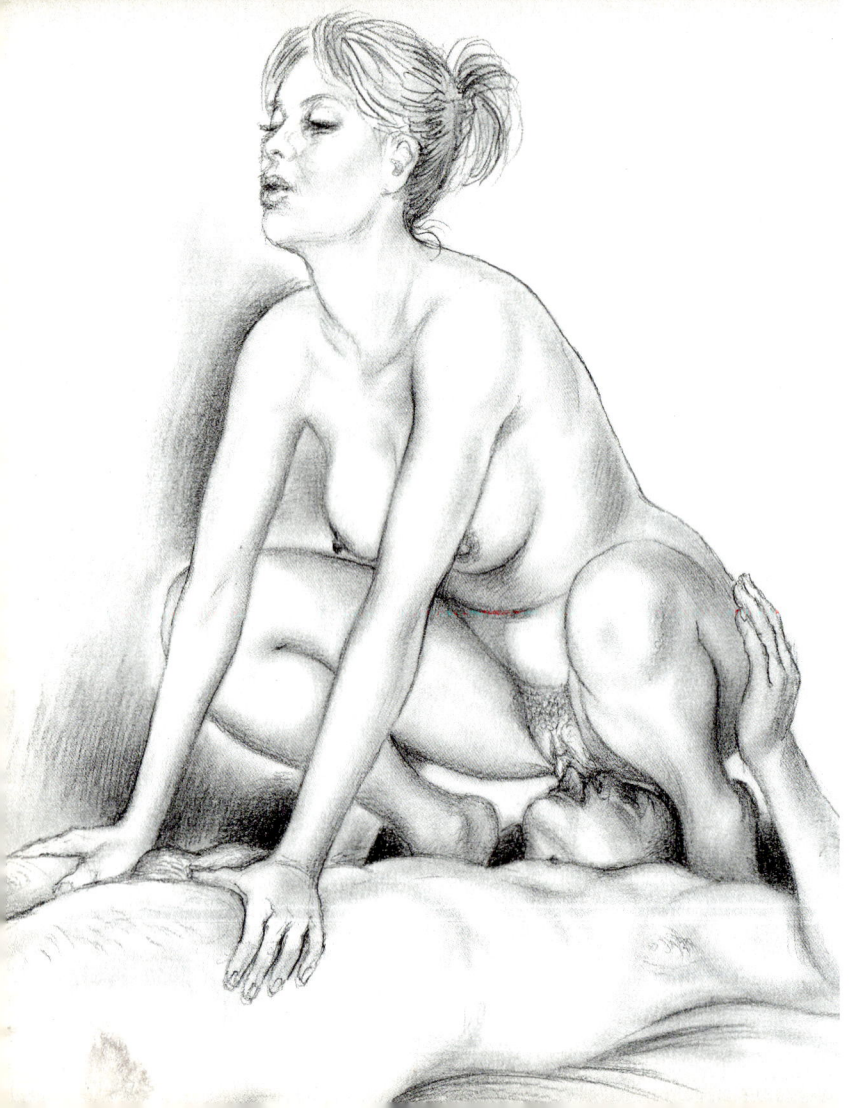

on her partner's thighs (but not the top of the knees), or wherever she wants. This will allow the cunnilinguist a bit of play, similar to that enjoyed in the "sixty-nine" position.

(3)   If there is an upholstered chair with padded arms or back to rest her knees on, the woman can present her vulva to her partner's face. The cunnilinguist can then support her legs as well.

Because these positions involve conscious choice and conscious agreement, there is very little way to avoid some "drama". Each participant has to express some kind of attitude to the other. Some kind of eye-contact, some kind of communication, which acknowledges their awareness of what they are doing.

There is, of course, the risk of embarrassment, in acknowledging and expressing feeling, but that embarrassment is a risk at all just

Face Sitting
(this page)
***Standing,
The Sofa***
(opposite)

goes to prove the existence of a mental landscape every bit as "hot" as having gotten naked and fooling around in the first place.

As in life, signals can get mixed, awkward moments can suddenly rear up without warning, and decisions reversed or changed ("Let's get in the shower instead"). Having some kind of idea or theme, however vague or even confused ("This is so hot I don't know what to do next") from which to depart or elaborate on is very definitely one of the foundation stones on which to build greater excitement. There is a feeling of freedom, of choice, even if that choice is to "let go."

There is one other position to consider in this regard, and that is…

3. Doggie
She gets on her hands and knees. There is no need to elaborate on the animal nature of the position: its

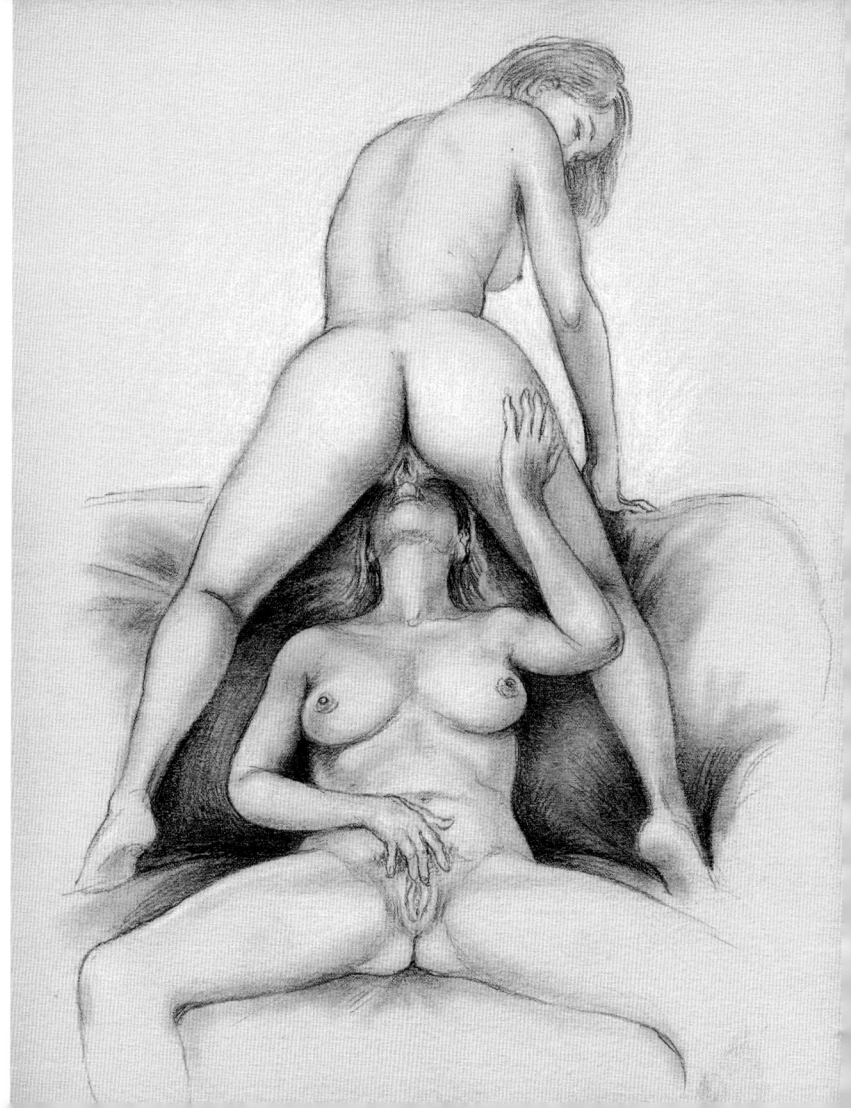

name says it all. Here is where the cunnilinguist's mouth and tongue are in play, but their freedom of movement is limited. However, this is where hands and other devices can really come into their own, either together or alternating with the mouth and tongue.

The fingers curl naturally downward; the G-spot is accessible, and two fingers can easily stroke on, or on either side of, the periurethral sponge. Orgasms in this position can be extremely intense, and the chances of copious ejaculation high.

Here is where dildos and vibrating dildos can be employed to great effect as alternatives to the mouth and tongue.

And Finally…

Of course there are many other positions, such as standing, vertical Sixty-Nine, etc. and various positions involving chairs or sofas.

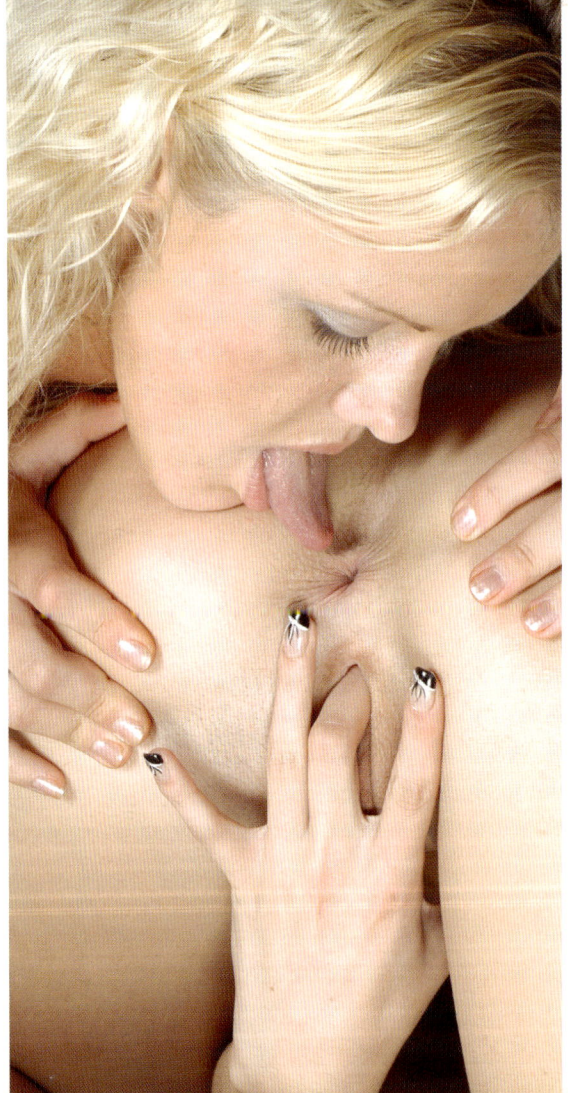

'Doggie' Position
(opposite)

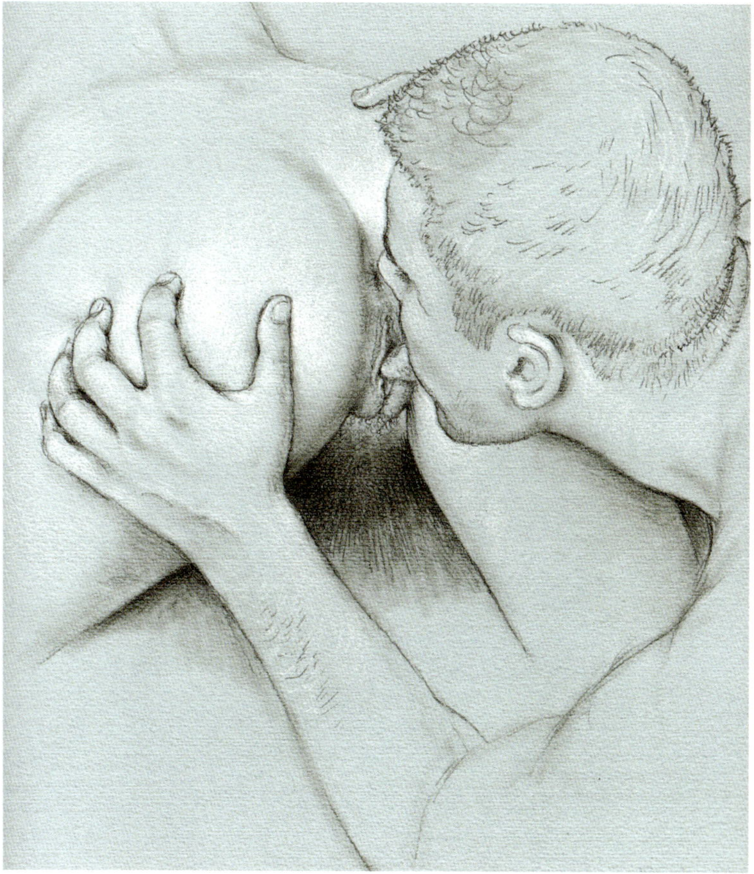

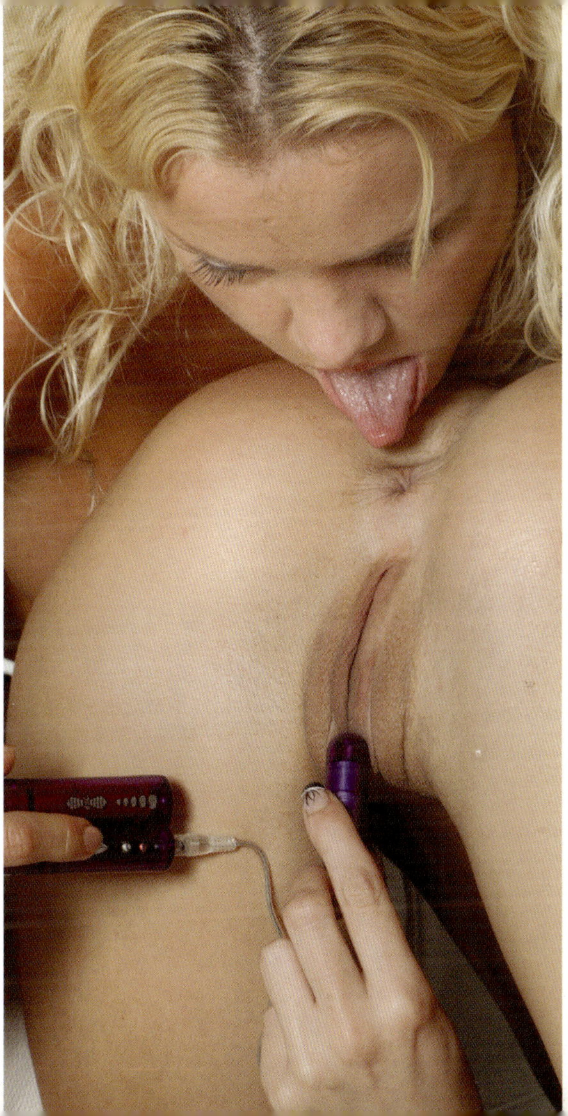

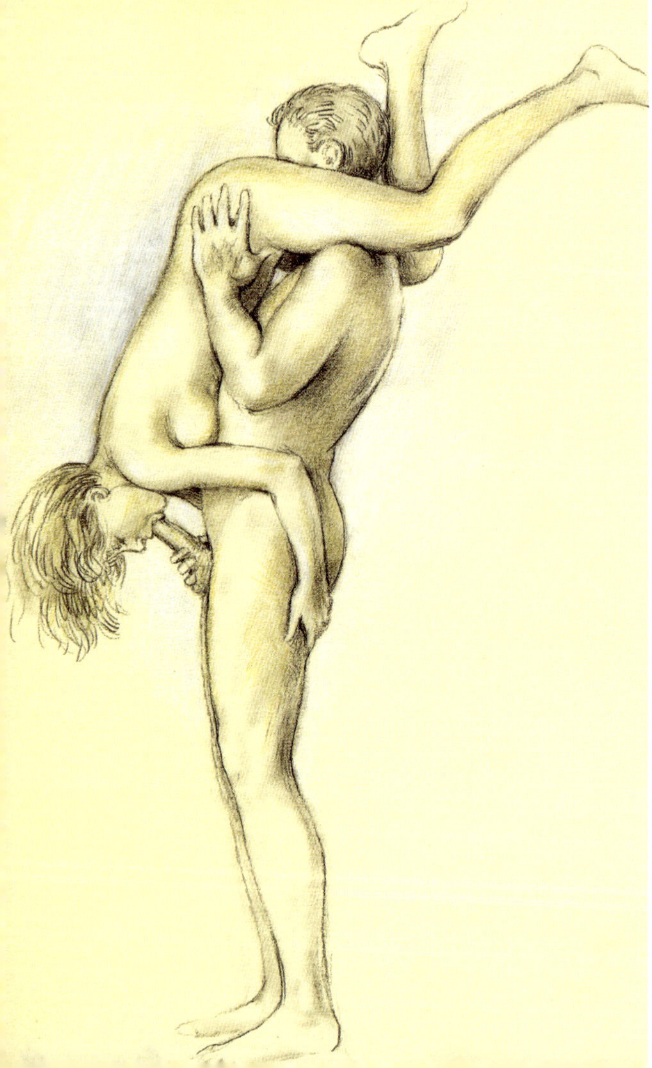

There is, clearly, enough left out to fill a book like this one many times over. But several important points must be made, however briefly:

The artful cunnilinguist does not have to display an entire panoply of techniques with each encounter, and should not be afraid of long periods of repetitive movements. Sometimes repeating a movement almost to the point of monotony is the very thing which can produce the most intense climax. What is important is that both participants are aware of whatever's going, and approve of it.

A great deal of emphasis has been given to the concept of tentative exploration, of gentle movement, of avoiding an 'ouch!' reaction at all costs! But this is more applicable to new partners, new situations, or special situations in a relationship.

Some women may complain about excessive sensitivity. More fool them. Concern for someone

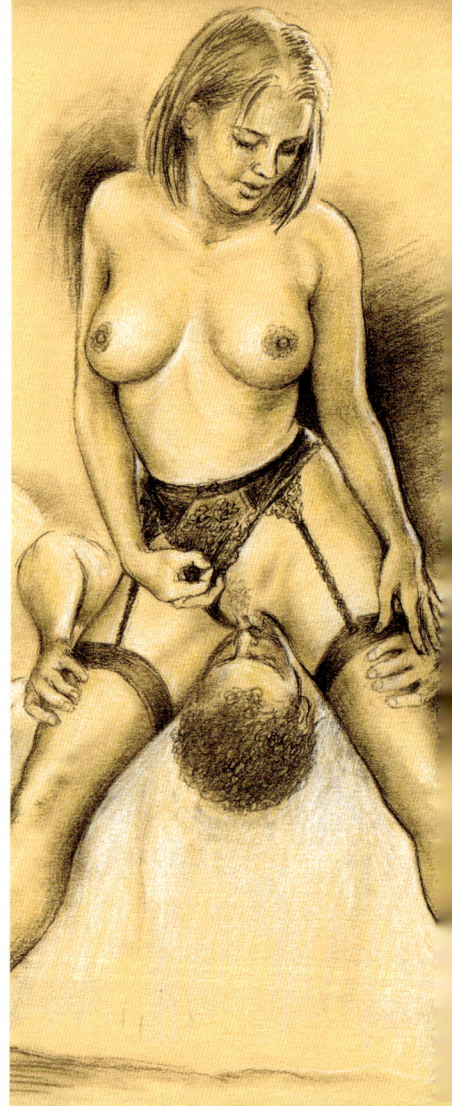

*Standing
(The Vertical
69)
Standing
(Bed)
(opposite)
Standing in
the Bath
(this page)*

else doesn't mean you're a "wuss." Sensitivity by the overwhelming majority of accounts is ultimately more memorable than showing off technique or "masterful control," regardless of whom one is with.

SO ROMANTIC

"My favourite time? We had just finished making love; we had both climaxed – me inside her; normally I don't like the taste of my come, but we were standing in the shower together and she gently pushed me down and my tongue roved over her wet breasts and nipples, her navel, bush and finally her pussy lips; I could taste the mixture of our juices and, to my amazement, found it was really quite delicious and very, very horny. I licked her to another orgasm and we just sank down and held each other while the water cascaded over us."

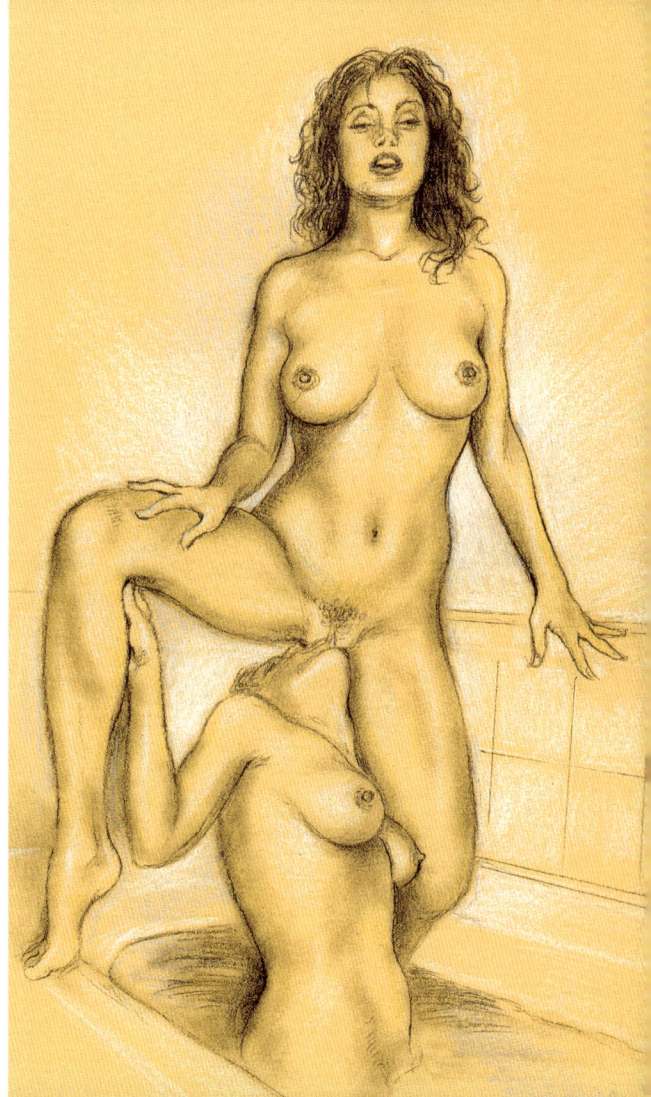

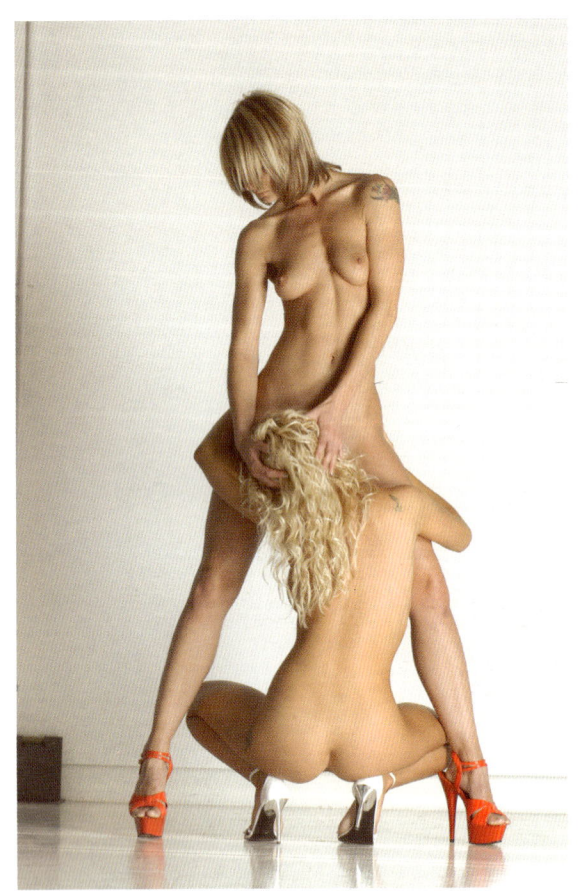
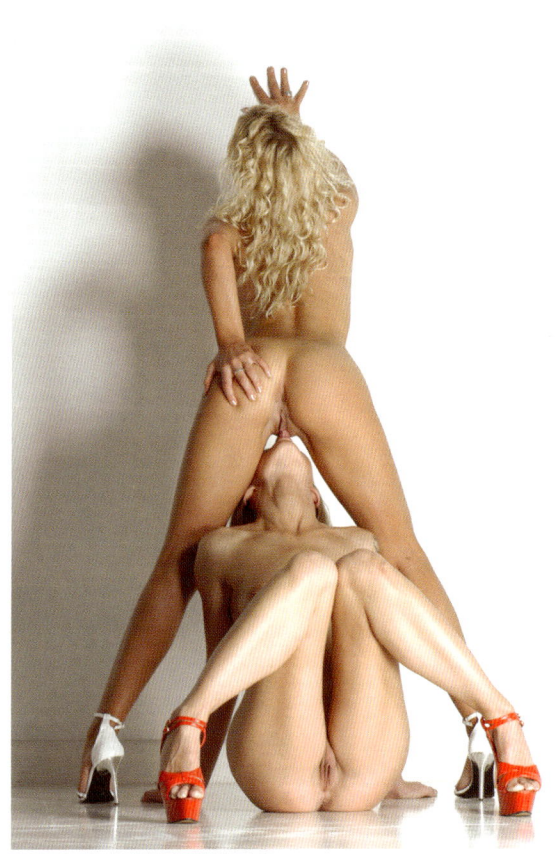

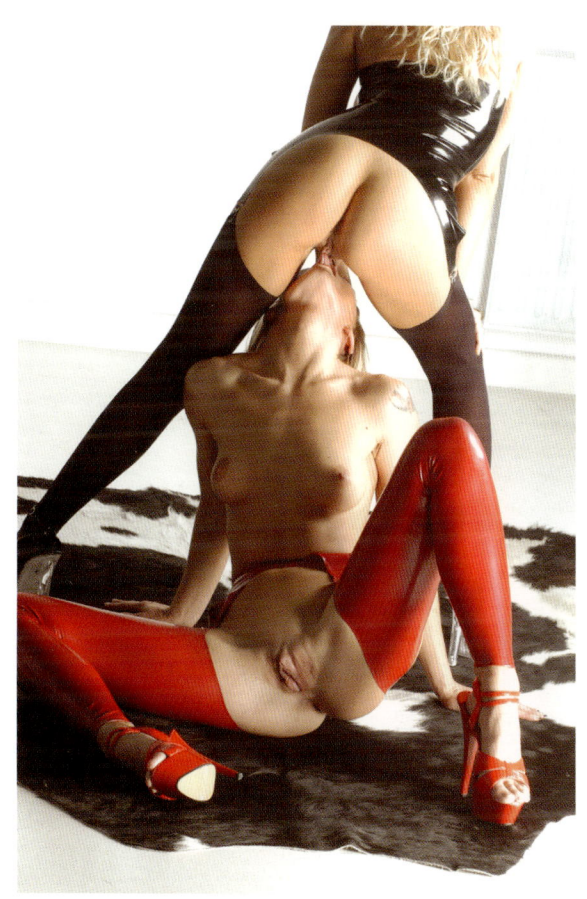
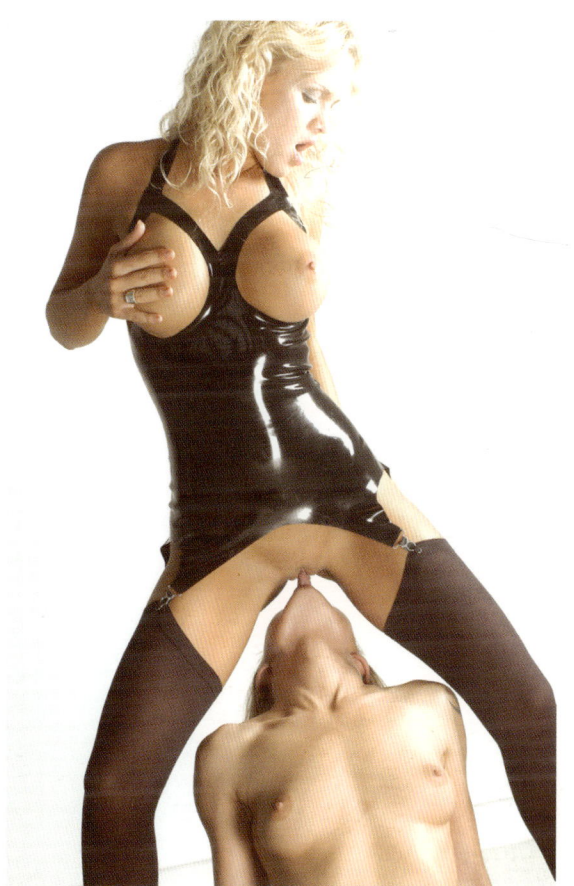

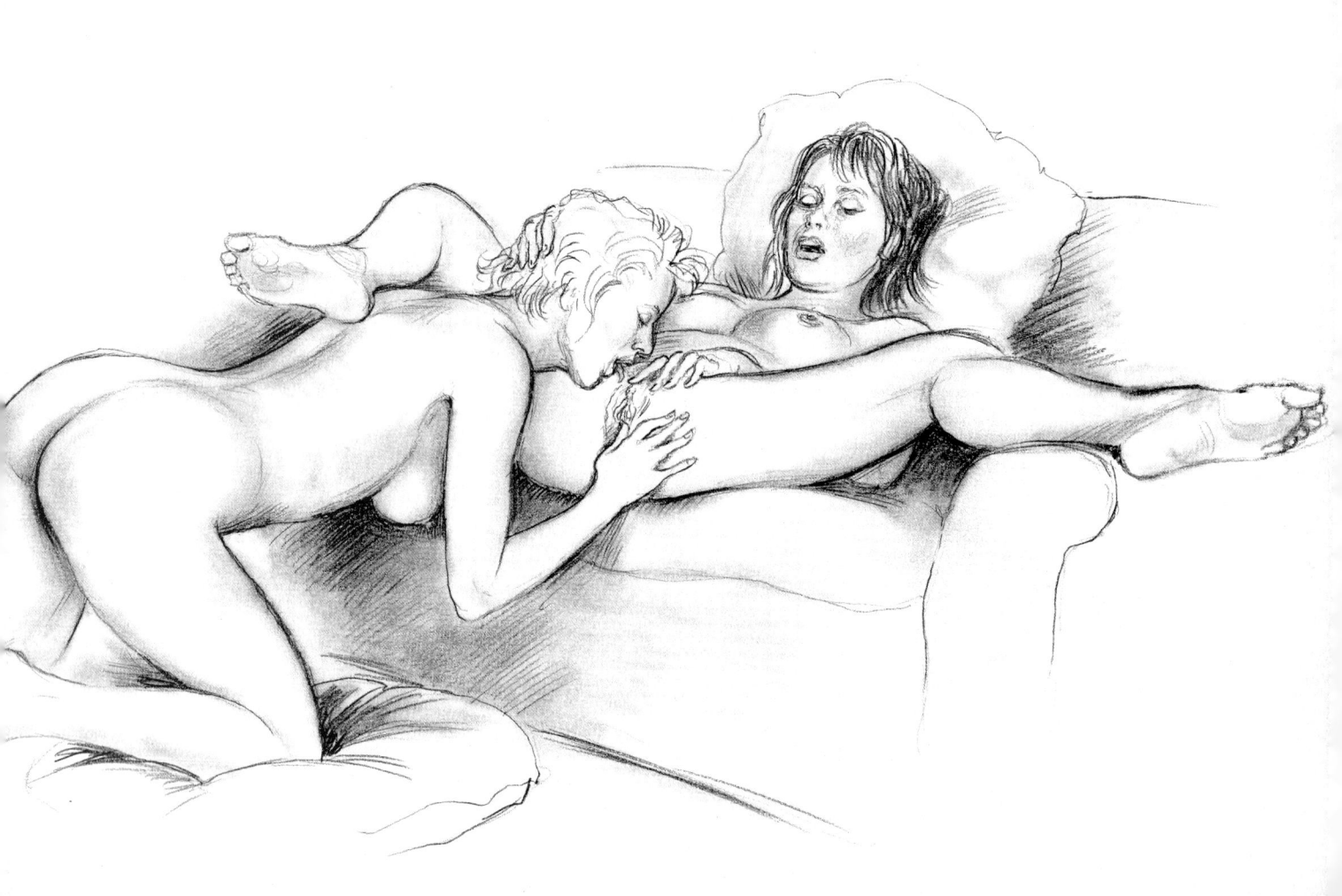

*The Chair,
Seated
The Chair,
Standing*
(this page)
The Sofa
(opposite)
The Chair
(page 90)

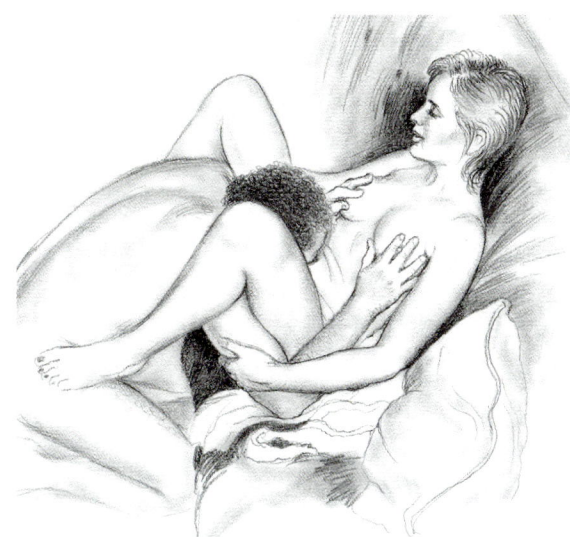

GO WITH A SWING

"My most interesting experience was when we were at a swinging party and our little group – there were five of us, three girls and two boys – made a daisy chain. Inevitably I found myself going down on my first woman, and later on the other two girls went down on me, which was another first. It was different, very gentle, intuitive and playful; although I'm not exactly a card-carrying bisexual now it's made me keep a very open mind about same-sex fun and games."

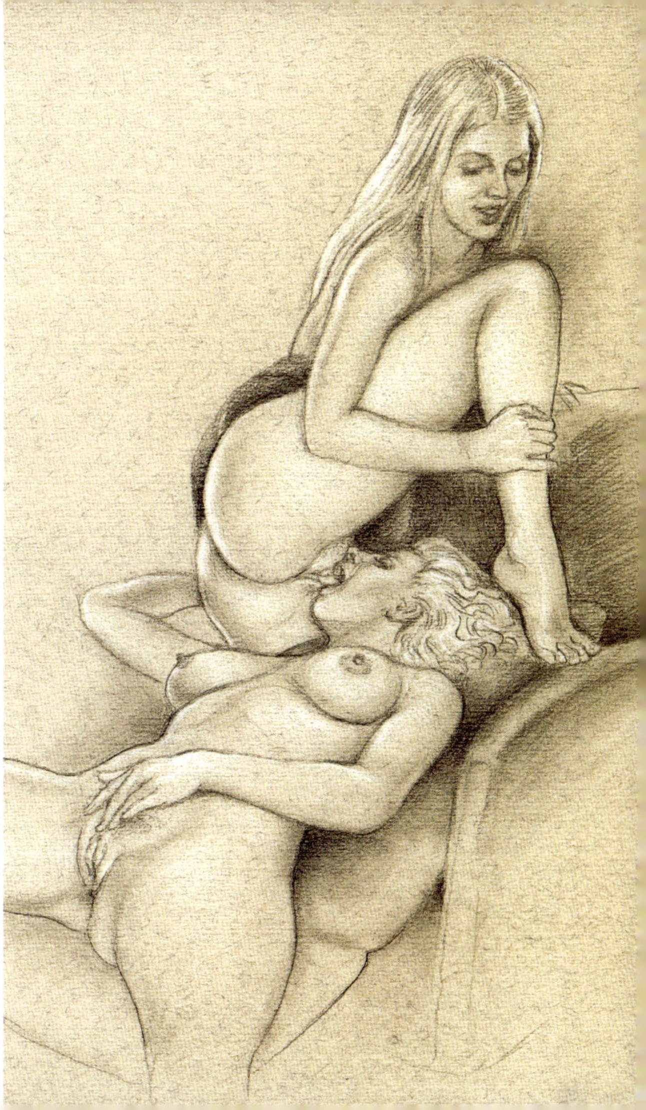

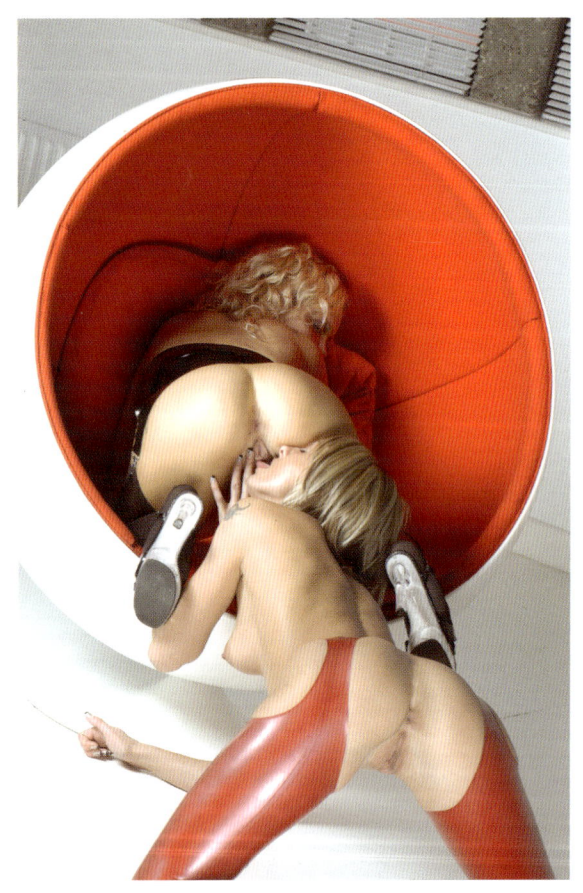
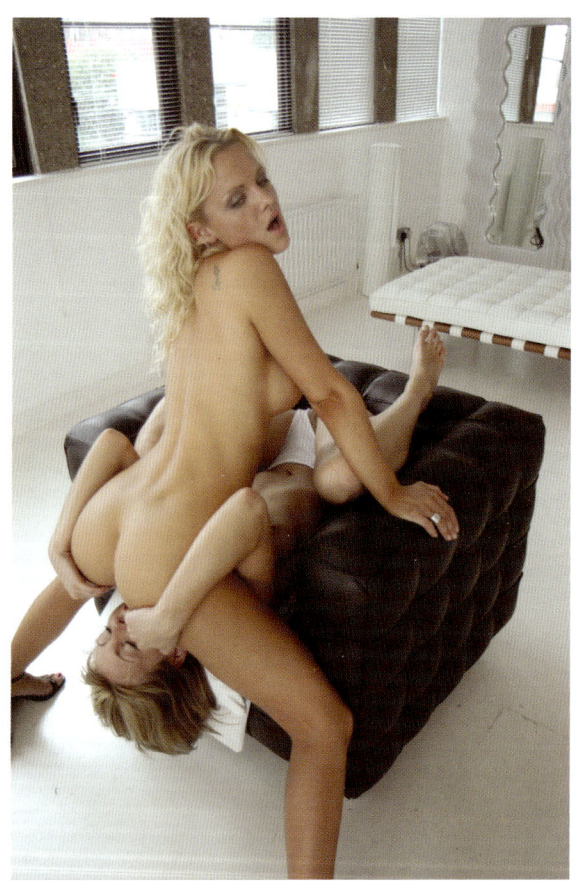

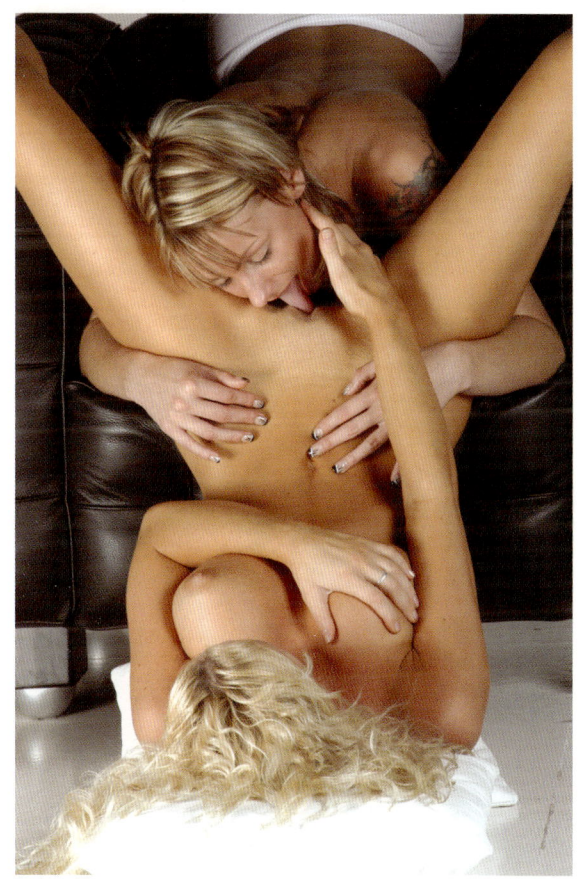
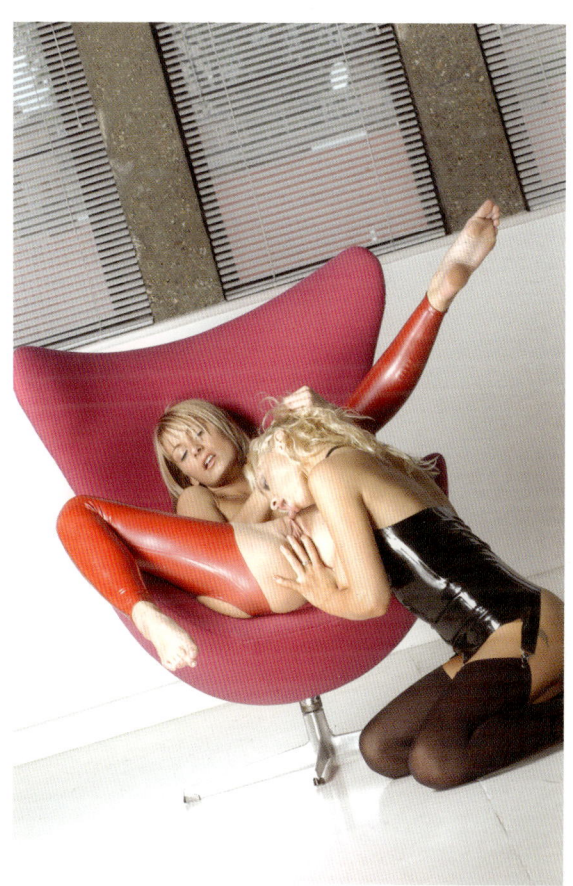

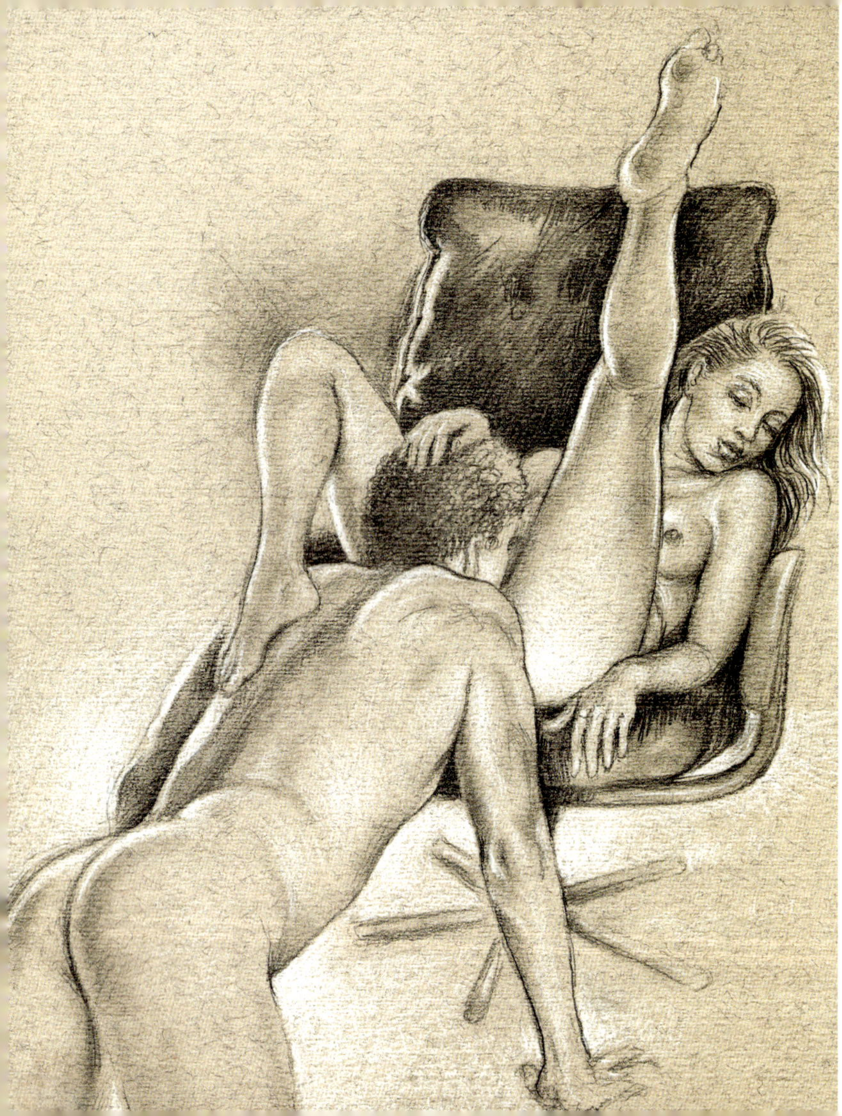

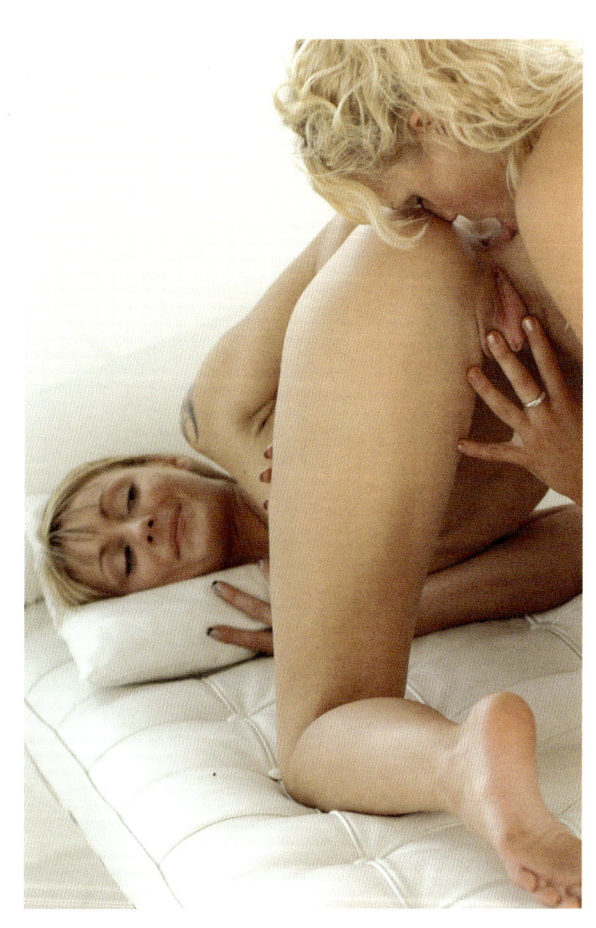

VII ABOUT HEALTH
& SOME BRIEF NOTES ON ANALINGUS

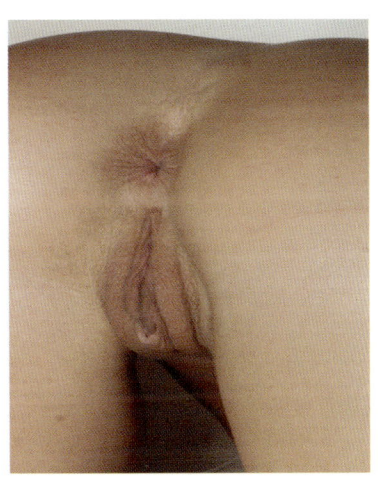
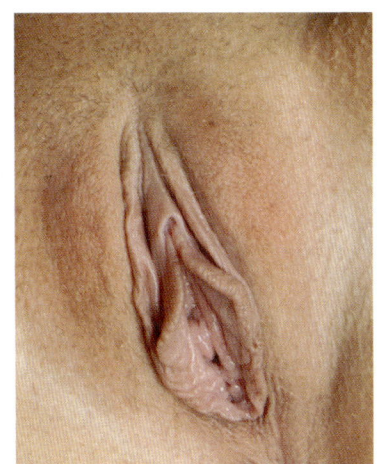

As this book is not for beginners, I will assume the reader is familiar with the dangers of the large number of Sexually Transmitted Diseases (STDs) around; that their incidence among the drunk, the over-trusting and the stupid are on the increase, and that there are simple precautions which can be taken to avoid them.

As far as cunnilingus is concerned, we only need post the reminder that:

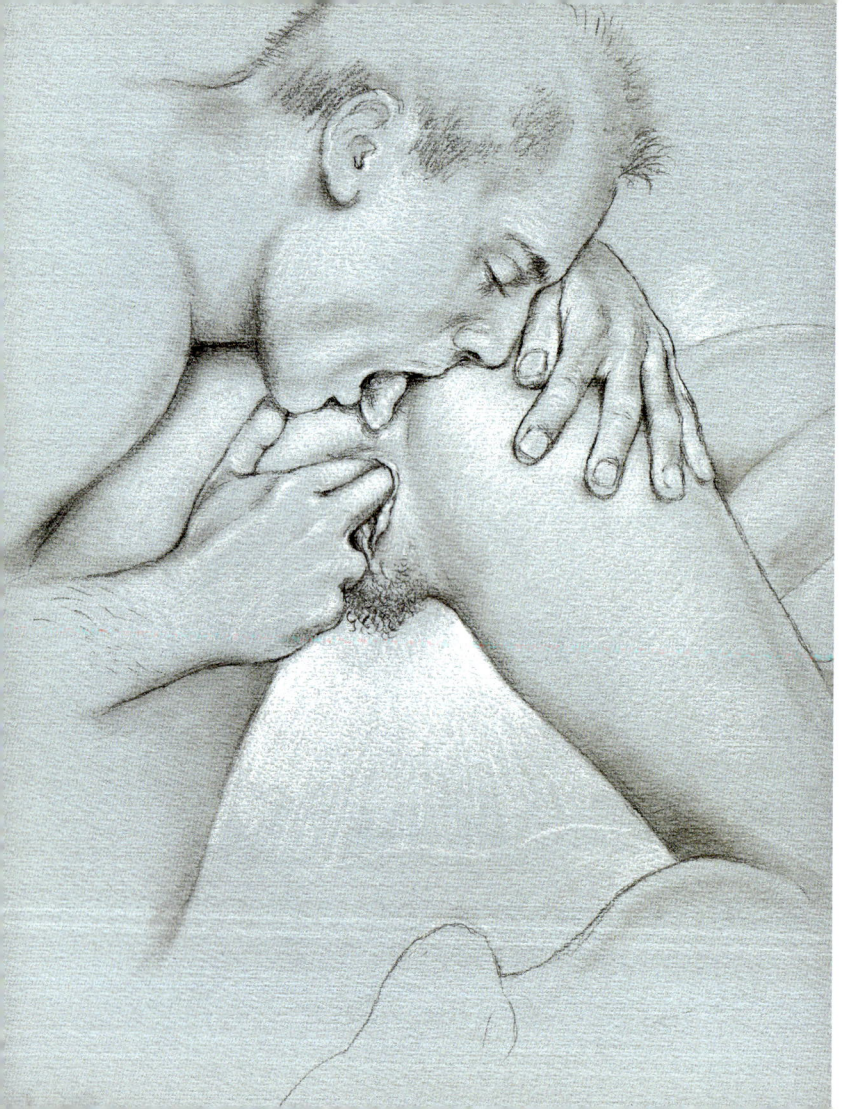

(1) condoms should be used on all sex toys (which should be scrupulously cleaned after each use in any case).

(2) all open sores, cuts, and ulcers mean that that area is susceptible to infection, as well as transmitting it, and should be avoided unless completely sealed by an impermeable barrier, such as non-microwave cling-film (good) or a dental dam (better).

(3) a good idea of your partner's sexual past as well as the scope of their present activity, establishing a mutual and well-founded trust on health issues and being transparently honest about any sexual adventures outside the partnership are all important factors in maintaining a healthy sex life.

Analingus with finger-play

HEALTH: BAD NEWS, GOOD NEWS

SEXUAL DISEASES are most often transmitted, perhaps not surprisingly, through unprotected sexual inter-course; unfortunately oral sex is no exception to the rule. You can still catch herpes (the genital variety can be transferred to the mouth and the oral variety to the genitals), AIDS (very rare), hepatitis B, syphillis, gonorrhoea, thrush and more, in this way. Dental dams, female condoms and non-microwave (the microwave stuff has small holes in it) clingfilm can be used as barriers against infection with various degrees of reduction in sensitivity, and you rather have to ask yourself the question - is 'protected' or 'barrier' cunnilingus really worth having? Unless there are exceptional circumstances, isn't it be better to wait until you are both positive enough about each other's sexual history and health to have full unprotected sex and feel secure about exchanging body fluids? But there are a few reasons as to why you might want to enjoy a bit of 'clingfilm' muff diving once you have established that you and your partner are 'safe': for the sheer kinky novelty of the experience (some suggest putting water-based lube on the pussy-contact side of the barrier for increased physical sensitivity), for genital ailments that, however temporary or minor are not things you want to share, and for oral sex during menstruation.

PERIOD MUFF

"I'm not wild about my guy going down on me when I have my period. I know it's silly, but I worry about the mess getting on the sheets and if we have to find an old towel or something it all seems a bit contrived. But when we're having a shower together it's fine!"

"It really doesn't worry me if Daniella has her period. I just think 'Oh, so it's that time of month, is it?' and get on with it. But a lot of my mates would rather die than do that."

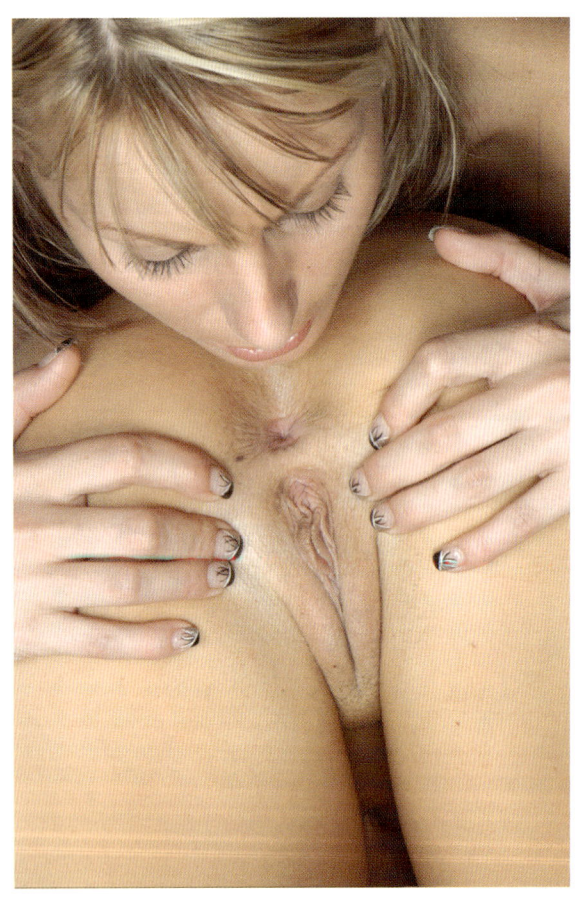

ANALINGUS: WHAT YOU NEED TO KNOW

ANALINGUS, OR RIMMING is when your partner tongues and licks your anus; strictly speaking, it's not within the scope of this book, but the proximity of the anus to the 'cunnus' is undeniable, so a brief mention seems sensible. Rimming is not everybody's idea of good, clean fun (early potty training may have rendered it a no-go area), but many who have overcome, or who never had, this particular taboo swear by it; the sensitivity of the anus is legendary and it's one of the few quasi-genital experiences that both sexes can share. Washing carefully is a must, but even so there is a risk of infection here (Hepatitis A, E coli and other bacterial infections, and intestinal parasites, for instance) and it's as well to be very sure of your partner's historic and current health. If you don't want to take any risks,

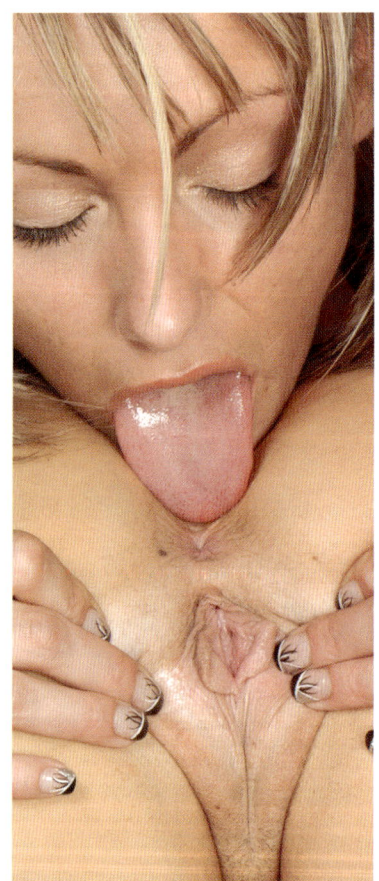

then get out the (non-microwave) clingfilm. A good starting point for analingus is in the shower so that preliminary hygiene (i.e. plenty of warm water and soap) can be effected to everyone's satisfaction before the act takes place.

With your partner face down, give her a back massage first, eventually arriving at her buttocks then gently parting them and kissing and licking them as you massage them too; gradually work your way in to the areas all around the anus: the crease above it, the perineum below it, and either side. She may want to hold her bottom open herself so that your fingers are free to stroke her labia and clitoris while your tongue is busy elsewhere. Then let your instincts take over and, using plenty of saliva, circle, probe, lick and lap the anal epicentre of sensation with your tongue. She'll love it.

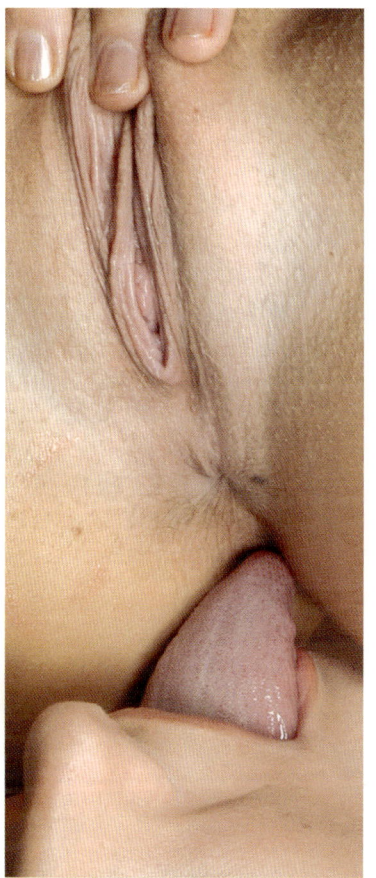

THE PLANET URANUS

"I love it when there's that moment of anticipation before he starts. The suspense builds and builds until his tongue is actual touching my anus; it's a great... no, the *best* prelude for full anal sex that I know."

"The first time that we ever tried it, it seemed very daring. Now we just do it occasionally for that wicked thrill that it always seems to deliver."

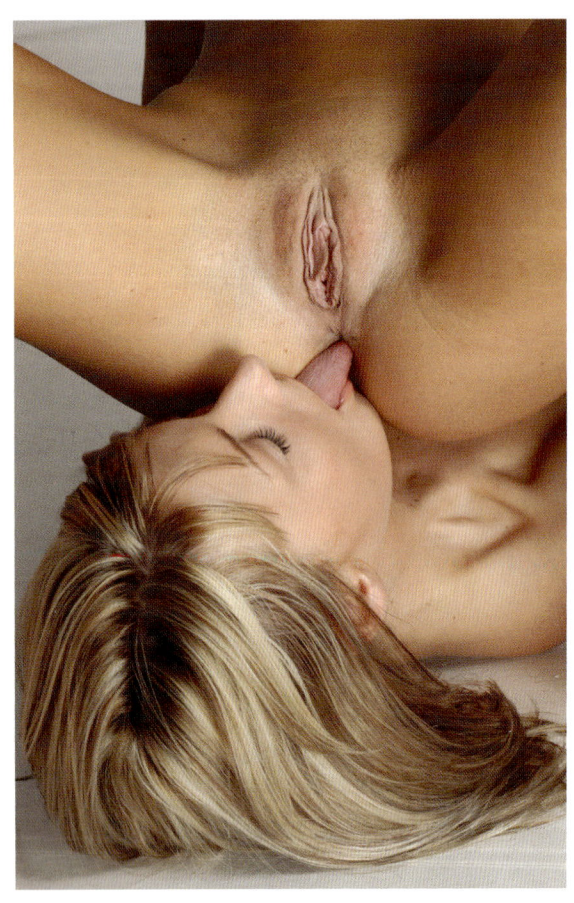

ANALINGUS: THE BEST POSITIONS

LYING DOWN. Always seems the most natural one – and good for when you've never done it before. Putting a pillow under her pelvis will give you much better access as her bottom will come up and the buttocks will part more easily.

KNEELING. This is a simple follow-on from lying down and gives the 'rimmee' more control.

'ANKLES BEHIND EARS'. Now on her back, she pulls her legs up until her bottom lifts off the surface to expose her anus. A pillow just below the small of the back is good here, too. For health reasons, DON'T be tempted to switch back and forth between anus and vulva; potentially it could cause infection.

STANDING. Interesting but tiring, and better access if the one standing has her leg raised, but liable to give you a crick in the neck. Sitting is better than crouching for the analinguist.

BEND OVER. A variation on standing. For those into mild S&M, this is potentially a favourite. Again, take a chair to it and sit rather than crouch or kneel. The rimmee needs the back of a sofa, a windowsill or the ledge of a box at the opera to lean over, especially during the closing, climactic moments.

'SIT ON MY FACE – PLEASE'. Perfect for the Dominatrix and her slave. She can look at your expression if she sits facing one way and if she sits the other, your degree of arousal (if you are male).

CONCLUSION

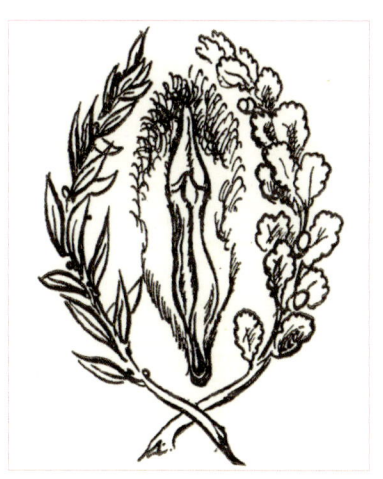 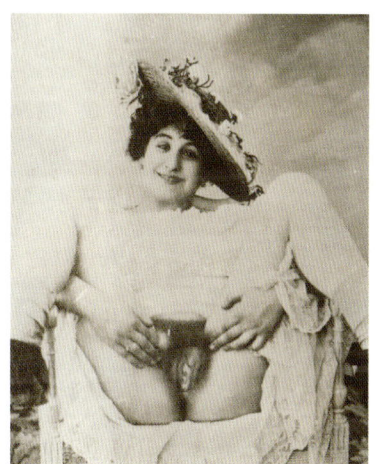

This book is a "Masterclass," however brief. It maintains the admittedly elitist idea that the "story-telling" aspect of cunnilingus, and by implication all sexual activity, increases sexual pleasure and distinguishes "story-telling", from mechanistic, sex.

Many people are terrified by the thought of not being sexually "spontaneous," which they equate with not being genuine, or "real", thus losing the "meaning" of the experience.

literature, often written by men for men (or by women for men), tends to eschew descriptions of cunnilingus altogether or, if it does refer to it, only fleetingly.

Artists similarly failed to warm to the theme, with a few noticeable exceptions: to make up for this lamentable dearth, here is a small portfolio of images by those who appreciate the true importance of the act.

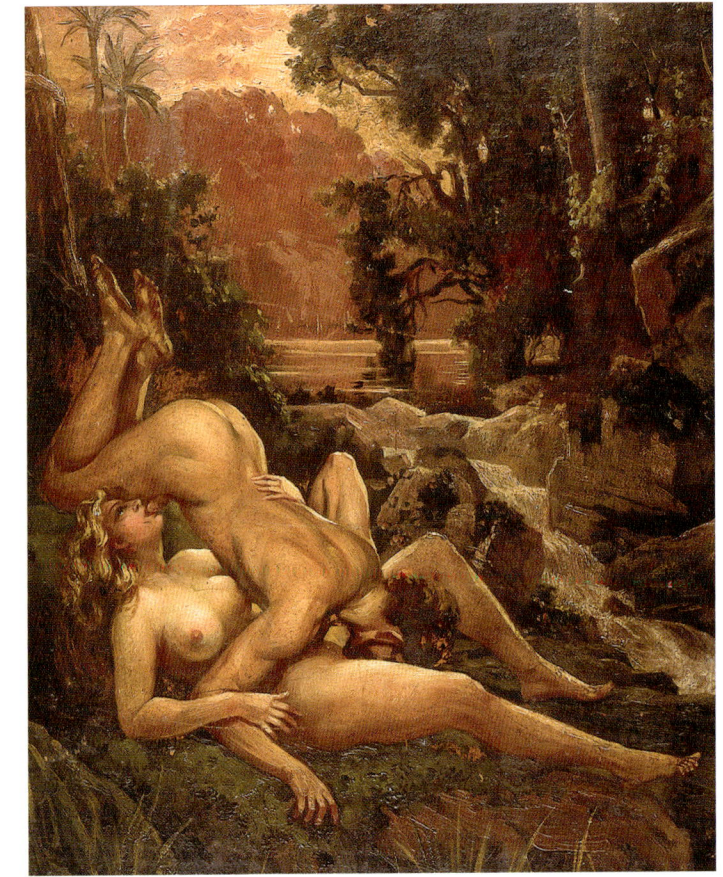

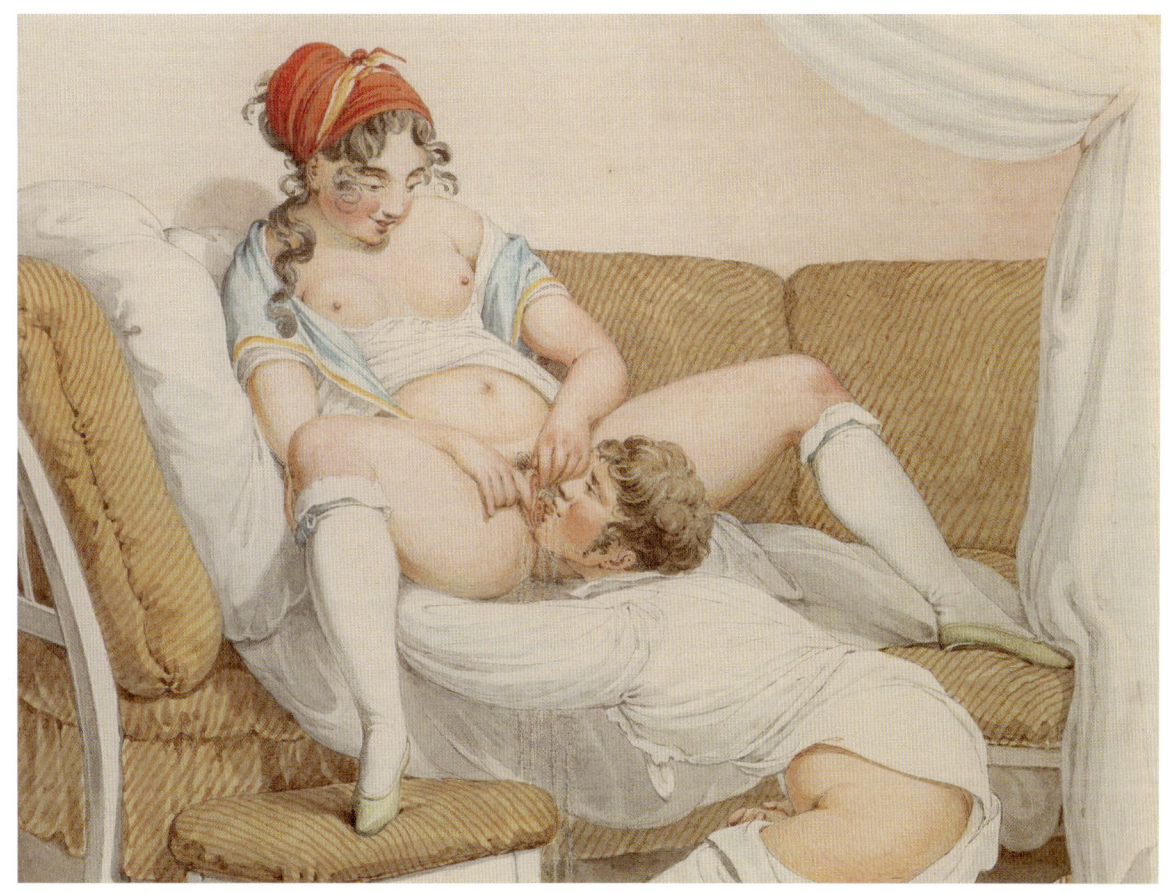

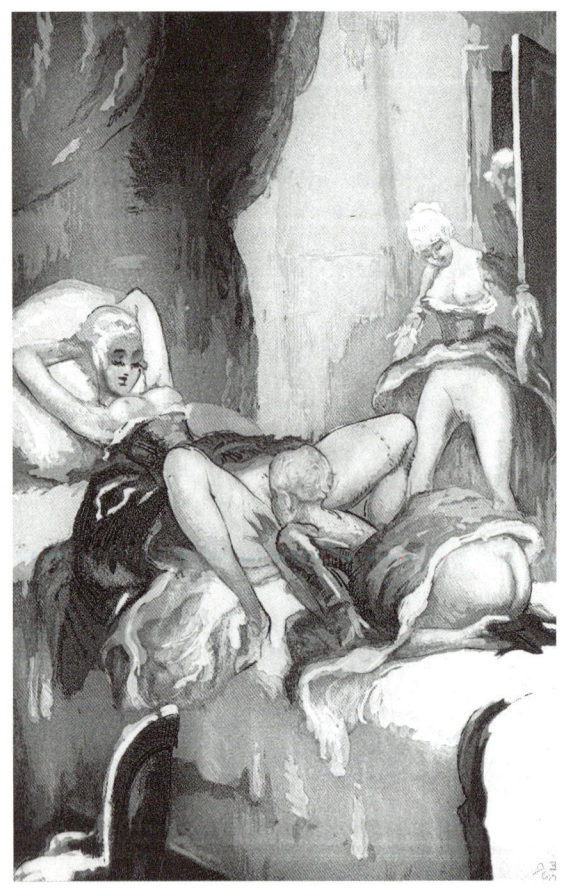
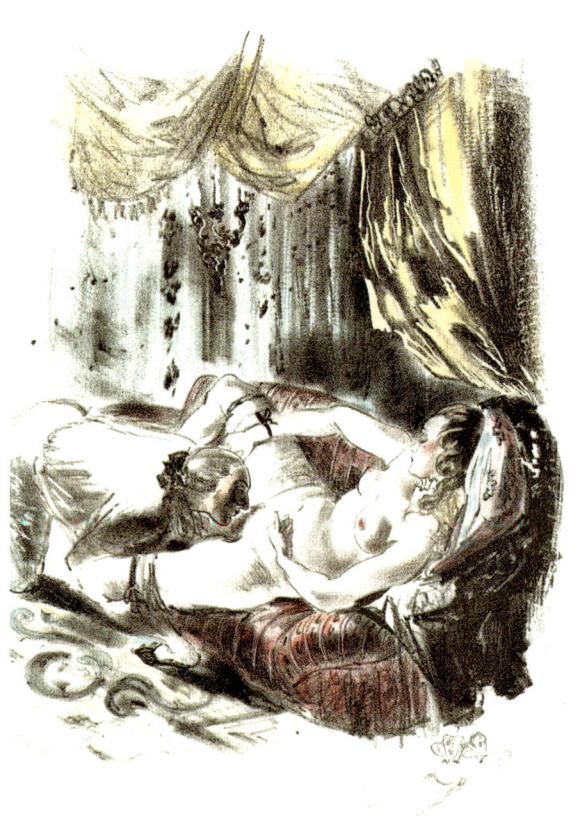

I succeeded in seizing the Countess' thighs firmly, and holding them wide open over my head. "Gamiani," I commanded, "come to me, a little further forward, supporting your weight on your arms." Gamiani understood what I wanted and I was able to enjoy running my agile and devouring tongue up and down her fiery slit to the utmost.

Countess Gamiani by Alfred de Musset

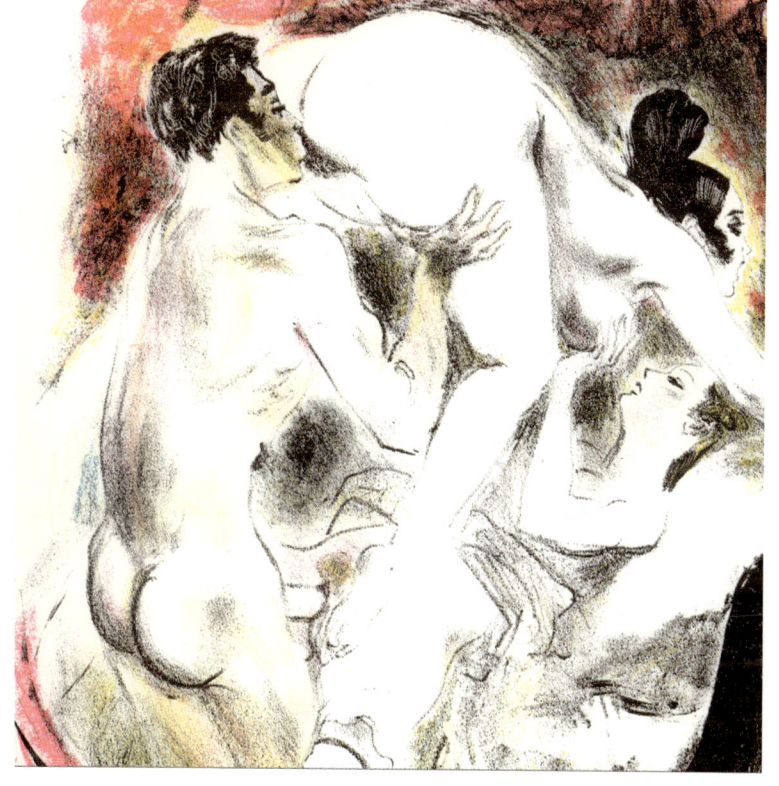

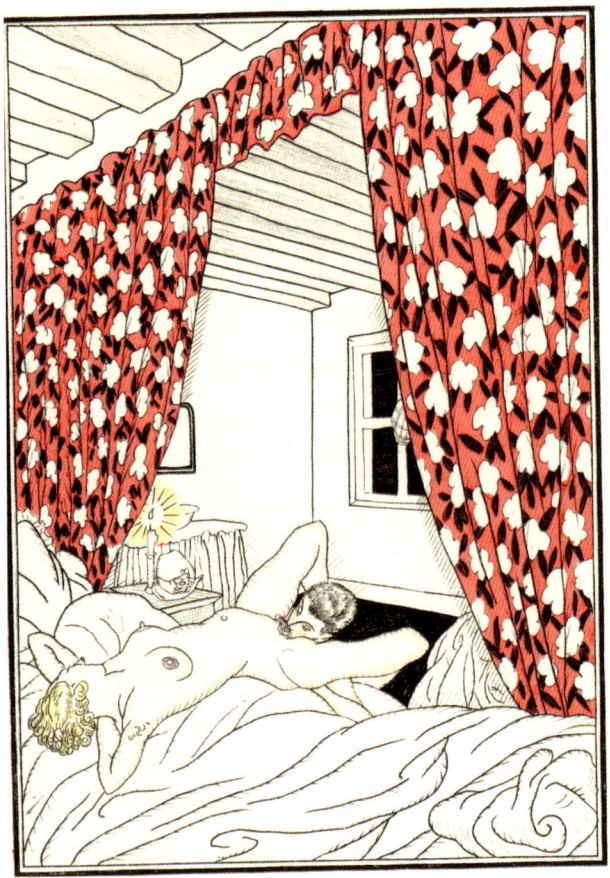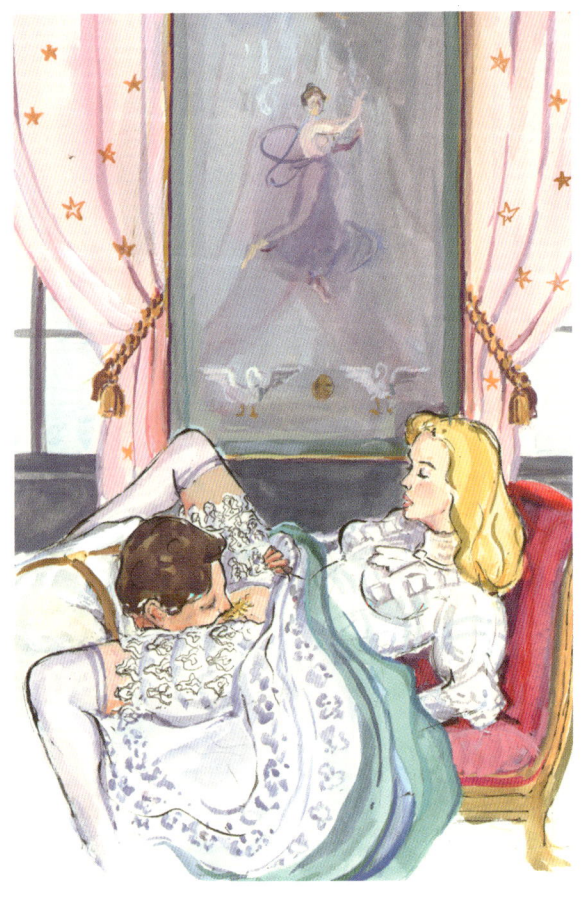

He parted her thighs with his two hands and avidly placed his mouth against the young girl's most intimate lips. He could feel the heat of her body; the usual odour, not at all unpleasant, emanated from the tiny slit which was extremely damp. He was just about to make Claire experience the spasm of love with his tongue when the marquis was heard turning the key in his door.

Séduction (anonymous)

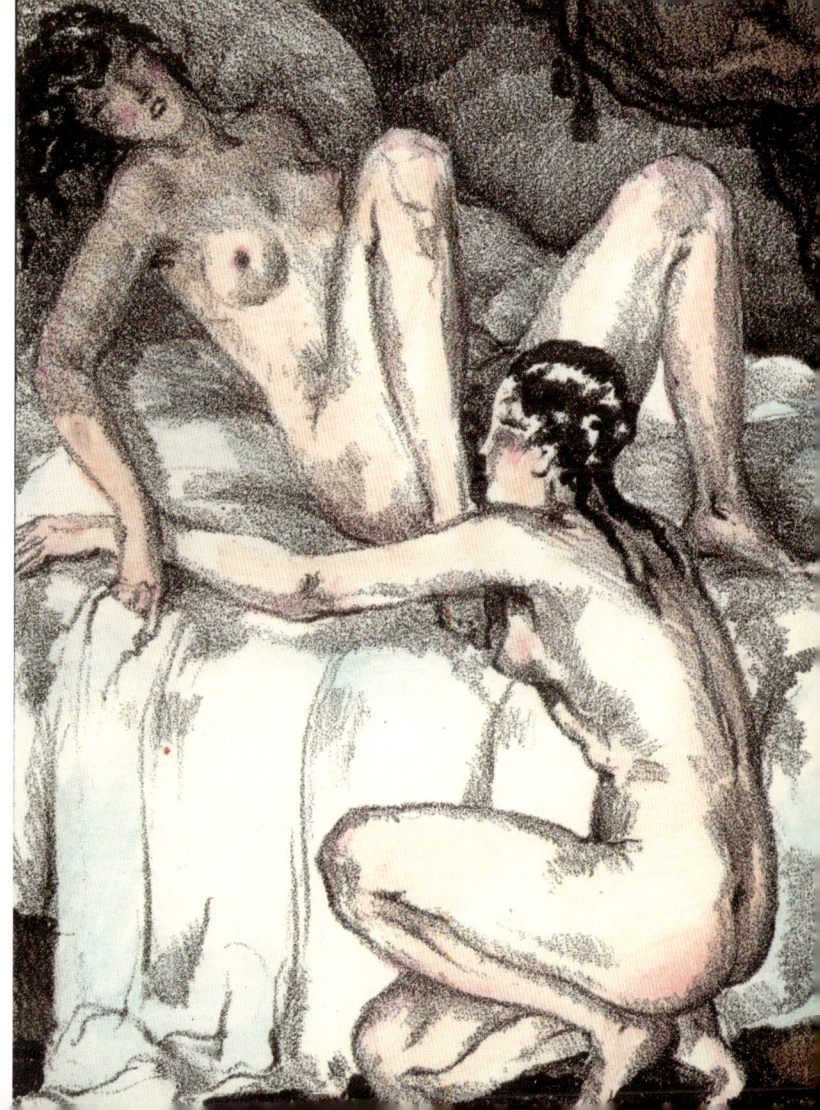

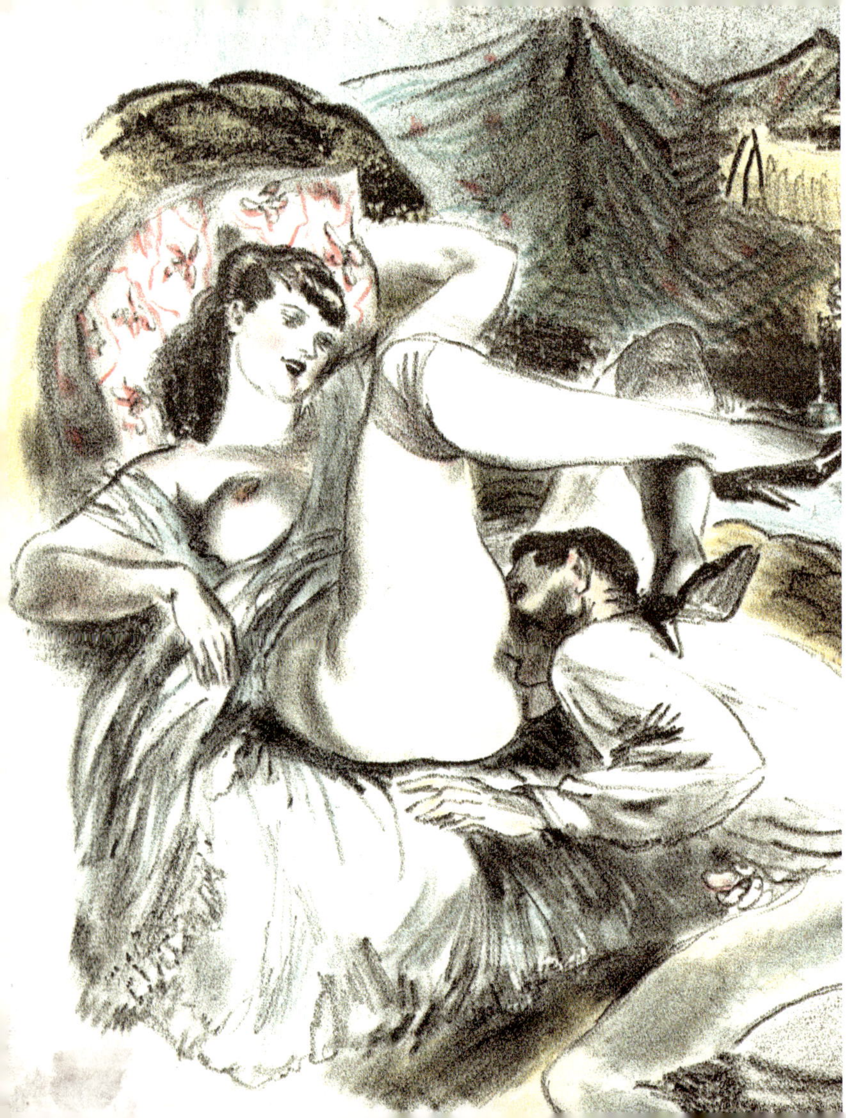

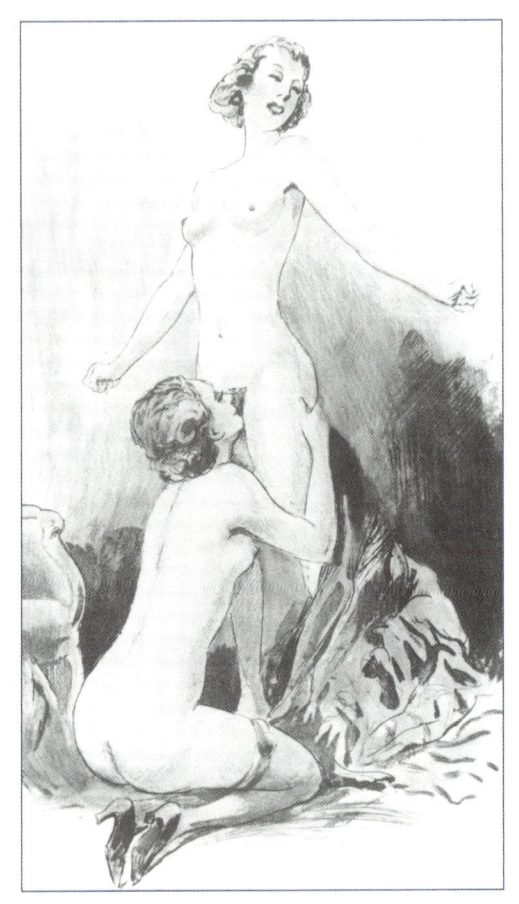

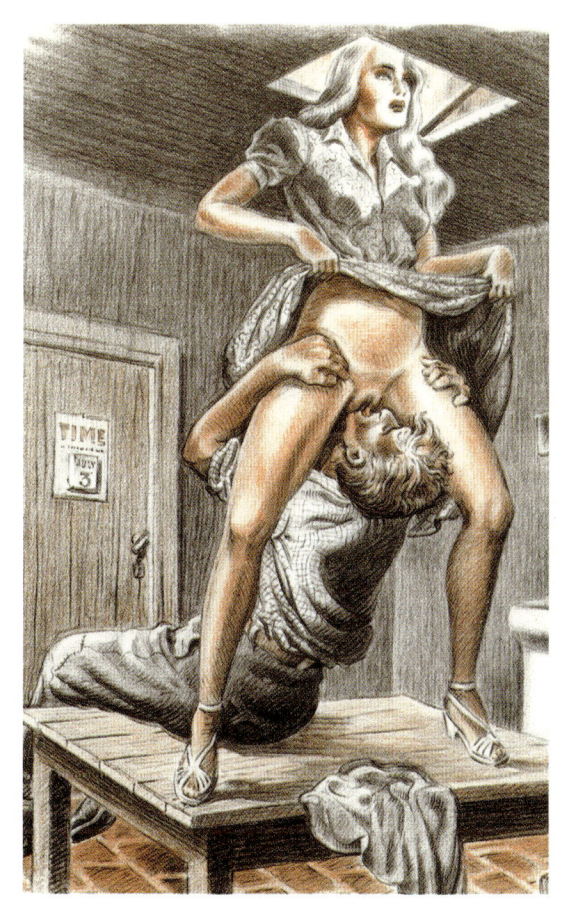

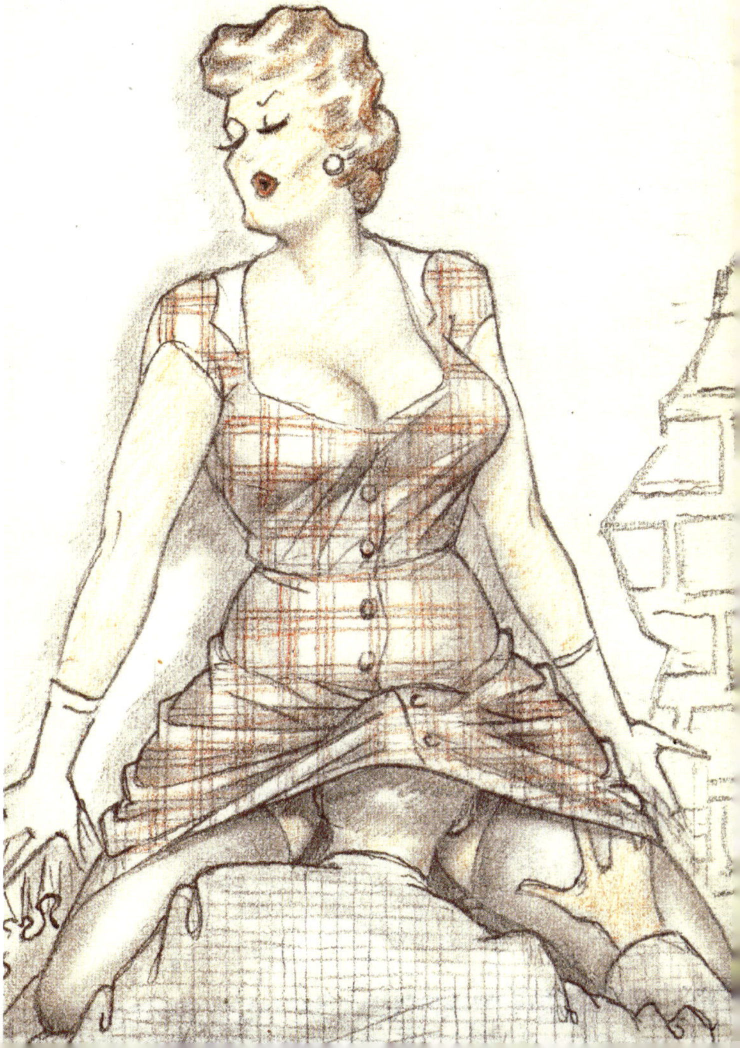

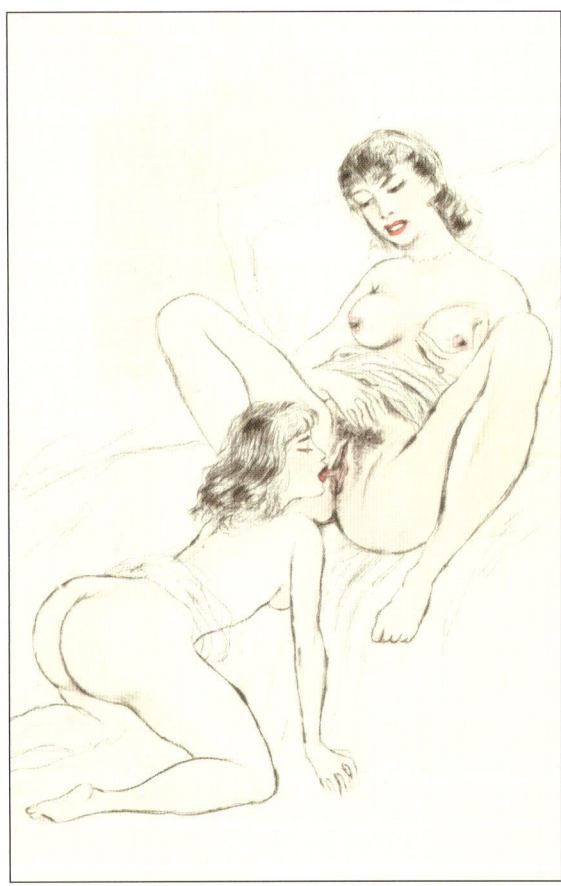

All pencil illustrations, page 20-92, by Lynn Paula Russell; all other illustrations from the EPS archives.

CUNNILINGUS
BY ANOTHER NAME:

CANNIBALISM
CHEW OUT
CUNT-LAPPING
DIVING INTO THE BUSHES
DOWNTOWN TO LUNCH
EATING AT THE Y
EATING FURPIE/HAIRPIE
FRENCHING
GAMMING
GOING DOWN ON
HONEY-POTTING
HOT DINNER
KIPPER FEAST
KISSING THE PINK
MOUTH MUSIC
MUFF-DIVING
MUFF-MUNCHING
MUFFING
PEARL-DIVING
PLATING
SIT ON MY FACE
SUCKING
TONGUING
WHISTLING IN THE DARK
YODELING IN THE CANYON

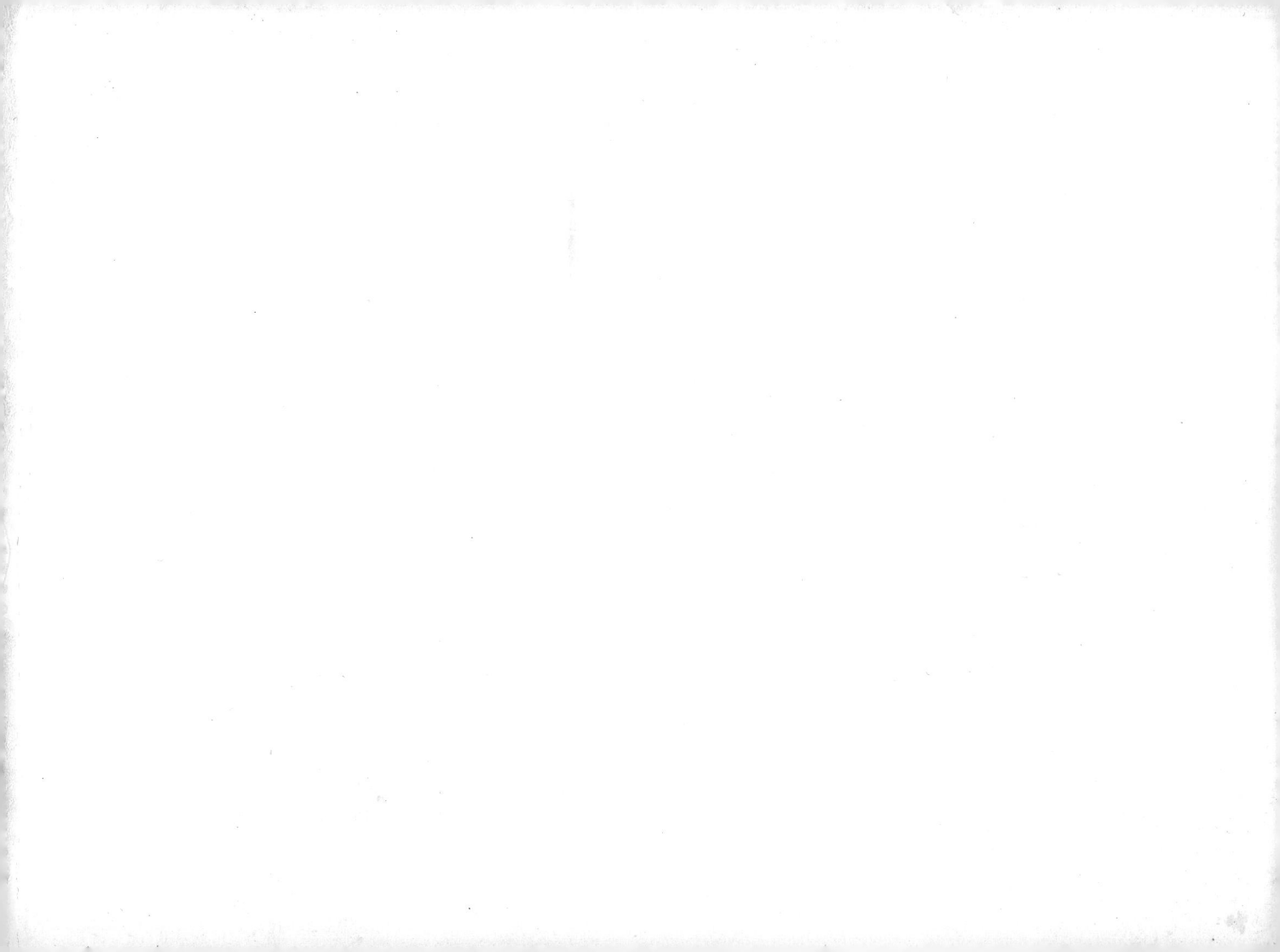